T0030520

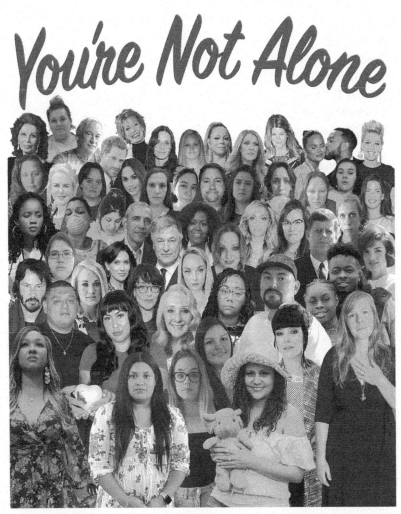

You're Not Alone

Shared Stories Of Pregnancy Loss

Michelle Fulton

You're Not Alone: Shared Stories of Pregnancy Loss

Published by:
Trine Day LLC
PO Box 577
Walterville, OR 97489
1-800-556-2012
www.TrineDay.com
trineday@icloud.com

Library of Congress Control Number: 2022945120

Fulton, Michelle,
You're Not Alone—1st ed.
p. cm.
Epub (ISBN-13) 978-1-63424-341-4
Trade Paper (ISBN-13) 978-1-63424-340-7
1. Bereavement. 2. Sorrow in parents. 3. Parental grief. 4. Mourning I. Title

First Edition
10 9 8 7 6 5 4 3 2 1

Printed in the USA
Distribution to the Trade by:
Independent Publishers Group (IPG)
814 North Franklin Street
Chicago, Illinois 60610
312.337.0747
www.ipgbook.com

Dedicated to:

Nathaniel Hendrikus Benningshof - Baby Benningshof - Baby Thalheimer - Baby Michal - Sofi Catherine Monney Siems - Sam James Simko - Angel Babies - Elijah James - Hiba Lael - Amelio Moses - Raymond Isaiah - Pumpkin King - Avery Jo - Jacob Anthony - Austin Chase - Alexis Jade - Bethany Grace - Aria Hope - Ivy - Ivan - Ivah - Baby Grigsby - Noah - Callum Jones - Addison Tess - Casey McDonald - Hannah Grace – Matthew Gulbrandson - Dakota Emilene - Scottlyn Grace Shank - Isabella Love Brodsky - Samuel Mark Isaiah Brodsky - Lynbrook Shalom Brodsky - Richard Cole Peterson - Matthais George Cruise - Asher Theodore Cruise - Genevieve Grace Cruise - Beloved - Esther Marie Jones - Haddy Ann Smith - Bruce N. Smith - Minnie Oletta - Everett Jacob Saenz - Franky James-Shiloh Ray - Alessi Eden Gulutz - Elizabeth Nicole - Isaac Leonard Hall - Charlotte Faye Willingham - Austyn Layne - Callan Luke - Hayden Oaklee Gill - Evelyn Grace - Story Rae Bartlett - Dakota Angel - Adele Nicole Brooks - Noah Jamison Broyles - Reiner - Jadyn Lehman - Jordyn Lehman - Jubilee Lehman - Isabell Grace Andersen - Faith Anderson - Kaulee Faith - Addisyn Grace - Kahara Prime-Kennedy Grace - Jessi Norton - Gabriel Matthew Mancini - Micah Henry Namjun Yoo - Lorelei McCallister - Robert James Comiskey - Calvary Grace Demes - Elijah Mathew Fortune - Shiloh Bennett Zolman - Hailey Elizabeth Marshall - Liath Umias Ventura - Sebastian Sterling - Emma Grace - Braeden Liam - Lauren Olivia - Owen Thomas - Hattie Luann - Luke Robert Hirsch - Ayla Grace - Jamie Robert Collins - Poppy Pip Tuttle - Gavin Paul - Kieran Buck - Sprout - Lihan Pretorius - Noela Mae Dickerson - Nasir Esai Jones - Ellie - Jaelyn Beck Howard - Amir Kay Giles - Zara Philip - Christian Philip - London - Autumn - Sydney Fazio - Laci Jo Hill - Lachlinn Allen Hill - Baby Witt - Caleesie Miracle Collins - Riemer - Ryan Michael Willhite - Sophia Grace Willhite - Ollie James Mefford - Baby Wells- Elouise Wells -Scout Wells-Ogden Wells - River Solace Hansen - Paisley - Brody - Carly - Maverik - Aubrey - Curtis - Elisha Osondu - Grant Ryan - Morgan Lee -Nora Jane-Baby E Estepp - Gideon Denver Bennett - Baby Tatum -Michael Ray Tatum - Declan Lawrence- Adeline Maire May - Isabella - Everleigh -Huntley - Angel Seagers - Jordan Seagears- Christian - Noel Seagears - Baby Seagears- Yani - Marigold Anne May - Oliver Forest -Noah Lewis - Avi Lee - Ruth - Bailey - Dakota - Roe Hart Bullock - Ammi Ruhamah Bullock - Jabez Warren Bullock - Asha Hope - Journey Raine - Sparkle - Diamond - Shiloh Jolene - Eve Spring - Jack Ryan - Austin Walters - Sam Walters - Hope Walters - Reign Walters - Baby Kerns - Natalie Annette Potter - Baby Potter - Baby Potter - Baby Huebner - Angel Avila - Kaliko - Kai - Abigail Junebug Rose Berlanga -Sawyer - Mary James - Matthew James - Jordan Peyton - River Lane - Avery Brooks - Dakota - Dallas - Sydney - Angel -Sophia Avery Mullis - Talitha Cumi Blount - David Michael Blount Jr. - Dililah Jane Buckely - Anastasia Nashira Long - Jack Greyson Long -Isaiah Brey -Hannah Elizabeth - Bethany Jean Mallard - Lael Shiann - Blake Amman - Riley Amman - Jordan Amman - Devin Amman - Kellett Samuel Quin - Analyssa Grace Comeau - Alexander John - Baby Davi - Koda lee Clendenin -Gideon Judah - August Baynx - Maisie Pearl - Kelsey Marie Jones - Gabriel Elijah Trunick - Baby Kitchens - Chase Matthew - Gabriel Lee McCorkle - Nicholas Anthony Diaz - Baby Follum - Corbyn Alexander - Baby Bojniewicz - Scarlett Rose - Collins Everly Doolittle - Laurel Rae - Solina Joylyn - Baby Chisum - Alexander Christopher B. - Evie Elizabeth B. - Savannah Margaret B. - Emmanuel Joseph Shepherd Bosserd - Samantha Rose Miye - Sophia Marie Miye - Jayde Elizabeth Miye - Amelia Grace - Micah - Bud - Kai Angel Linares - Avery Linares - Rowen Dawn - Matthais Eugene - Aurora Jade - Jacob Anthony Gillette - Luke Alexander Garcia - Alaric Puentes - Atticus Puentes - Riley Lou Devins - Evelyn Elizabeth Ballard - Isaac Elisha, Odelia Rose, Anthony Matthias, David Andrew, Marigold Faith, Selah Abigail Whited - Brighton - Selah - Jesse - Devin Jobst - R.J. Swope - Remy - Jake Allen - Decker Babies - Eleanor Springer - Bailey Noel - Angel Perry - Silas Neveah - Kylie Addison - Justin Addison - Samuel Black - Amelia Rose Patterson - Angel Faith Boggs - Hope Faith Boggs - Aiden Kyle Boggs - Meira Bode - Brynn Bode - Bode Babies - Anglel - Devan - Jaramiah Oliver - Baby Jesse Jacobson - Baby Tom Smith – Isabelle Joy - Unnamed

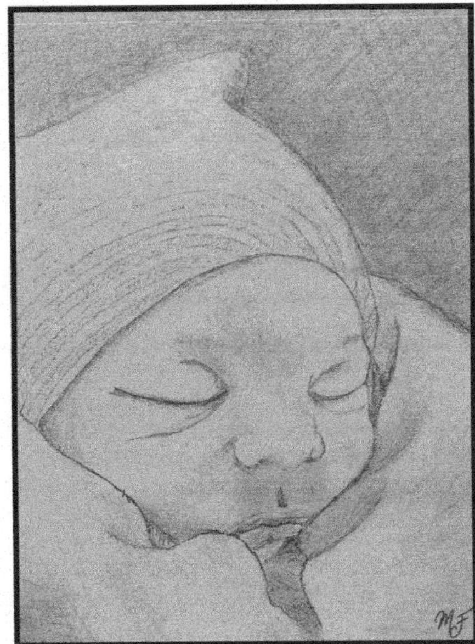

Inspired by
Cole Vaugh Taylor Fulton
and Leifje Benningshof
and
In Loving Memory of All the
Precious Babies, Named and Unnamed,
That Live Forever in Our Hearts.

INTRODUCTION

This may be hard to read, it may bring back difficult memories of your own experience, or your own experience may be so raw and fresh that it resonates with you on a soul-shattering level ... but I want you to cry. If you have experienced this in the past, I want it to free you to share your tragedy with others, and pave the way for open discussion. Be a pioneer, leading others to find comfort in community rather than solitude in isolation. And, my heart, if you have carried the burden of this grief recently, I want you to cry your eyes out, because tears release stress hormones and toxins, and they help soothe you by prompting the production of oxytocin and endorphins which can assuage emotional pain that could otherwise manifest in fatigue, physical pain, and continued depression. I want you to let the misery and tragedy of your situation wash over you. I want you to cry until you have no tears left because that is what helped me, and I believe wholeheartedly that it will help you too.

The following stories were contributed by mothers and fathers, from all walks of life, from all over the world, who have experienced pregnancy loss. You are not alone or isolated in your experience. Somewhere, someone knows how you feel, because they have been through something similar to what you have been through. You do not need to suffer in silence or solitude; know that there are many who understand and who can be there to support you as you grieve and come to terms with who you are now and where your life will go from here.

Take a deep breath. Take another.

You are not alone.

Contents

Introduction v

Foreword: We Are One in Four – by Danielle Muze 1

1) My Baby Girl by Debbie Martin 3

2) Pip's Story by Rose Skillcorn 7

3) Young Love by Luci Sorgiovanni 12

4) Waiting on a Rainbow by Jessica Oberlin 15

5) Joy in the Mourning by Tabitha Saunders 18

6) Broken to Blessed by Kayla Jones 21

7) Why, God? by Amanda Wong Loi Sing 28

8) Never Forgotten by Chelle Collins 31

9) Getting to My Rainbows by Natasha Pandeli-Veyssiere 35

10) My Journey to Motherhood by Dana Colon 42

11) My First Homebirth by Bee Portillo 44

12) God's Miracles – A Father's Perspective by Sergio Portillo Jr. 47

13) The Story of Our Angel Babies by Katie Lee 51

14) Zoe Grace by Alana Zoufal 58

15) Three Butterflies by Y. Jordan 69

16) Nathalia's Purpose by Dina Mejia 78

17) Quarantine Losses by Ms. Khat-Eyes 91

18) Remember Me, Rain by Hailey Shields 96

19) My Angel in Heaven by Tammy Nichols-Rogers 101

20) Whispers of Comfort by Dee-Anna Janku, ... 103

21) Alexander Rodriguez by Silvia Rodriguez 107

22) Declan and Devlan by Marsha Sparks 112

23) A Letter to My Angels by Justina Engen 116

24) Two Little Lights by Peter Wright 128
24) You Were the Best Thing I Ever Knew I Needed, My Prince by Lauren Kirwin 132
26) Healing from Loss by Eze Modester 137
27) Jennifer's Story by Jennifer Coulter 140
28) My Sweet Althea by Kelsey Kirkpatrick 153
29) My Son I Couldn't Keep by Laura Ebel 157
30) Losing Anna by Sarah Khouri 160
31) Reclaiming Your Identity After Stillbirth by Jessica Tamez 163
32) Touched by an Angel by Trinity Brown 165
33) Losing My Daughter by Janel Neff 167
34) Goodbye Before Hello by Melissa Ziegler 170
35) The Light in the Dark by Dustie Euler 178
36) Through the Eyes of a Father by Ed Hamilton 185
37) You Will Never Have a Cloudless Sky but the Sun Will Shine Again by Daniel Harding 192
38) The Life of Emory by Sunshine Penny 198
39) I Had a Son by Michelle Fulton 202
40) Remembering My Samuel by Rachel Wheeler 221
41) Adrian's Story by Miranda Hernandez 224
42) Letter to Reader by Kristine Bernadette C. Millanar 229
Acknowledgements 231
You're Not Alone Resource List 233
Index 239

Foreword

WE ARE ONE IN FOUR

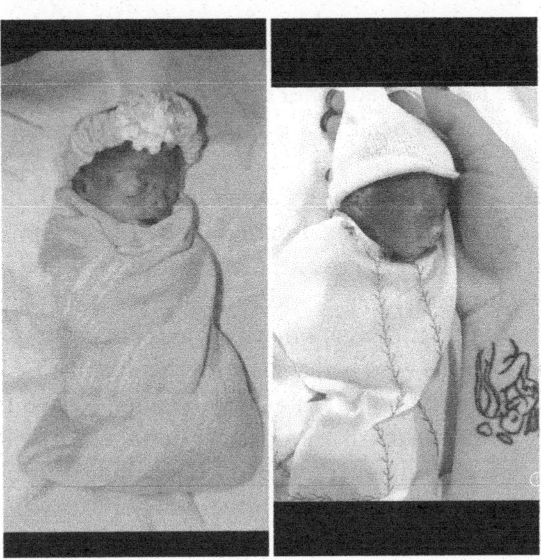

By Danielle Muzer

I am here for you; I am with you; we are one, all together. You are not alone, and you will never be alone. Losing a baby at any stage (whether by miscarriage, preterm labor, or even stillbirth) gives you the right to feel how you feel.

I have experienced two pregnancy losses within a two-year period. My first loss was on January 14, 2018, at twenty-five weeks. My beautiful baby girl, Addison Elizabeth, arrived too early due to preterm labor. Although she was at a viable stage, she did not survive. My second loss was at twenty weeks, on December 21, 2019. My handsome son, Logan, also arrived too early due to preterm labor. That day, I was diagnosed with an incompetent cervix.

This was a very tough journey for me, and it will be for you as well. You will feel anger, you will feel guilty, you will feel like you're not good enough to be a mother or father, and you will feel SAD. All of this is normal, and I want you to know that you are not alone.

Going through something like this, that is so traumatizing, really changes your whole perspective of life. My main struggle was coping with whether this was a bad nightmare or my reality. The truth is, this life-challenge is both. There are highs and lows; I call this grief a roller coaster.

You will have really good days and really bad days. Some days you will love seeing babies and kids, and other days you will cry just from seeing them at the store or scrolling through social media.

After my first loss, my best coping mechanism was writing, writing how I felt. It feels so good to just write how you feel, especially if you have a hard time talking about what's going through your head. I tried counseling but I felt like no one could ever understand and help me if they had never been through the same loss as I had. After my second loss, I finally sought counseling. I wanted to find a healthy way to cope with grief instead of burying it inside my heart.

After my second loss, the best coping mechanism for me was helping others who had also lost a baby. I ended up being an administrator for a pregnancy and infant loss group and many people reached out. It was like one big family who truly understood each other. I didn't know how common this was until that moment when I joined that group; there were way over one-million people who had lost a baby just like me ... just like you.

Your days will get better, brighter, and happier. No, you will never get over this, but I promise you that it does get better. Take one day at a time and see how you feel, and never feel bad for reaching out to someone. Do not feel ashamed. We are all in this together – we always will be for the rest of our crazy life-journey. There is so much love in the baby-loss community that it could light a million stars. I got this, you got this, we got this.

Much love,
Danielle

1

My Baby Girl

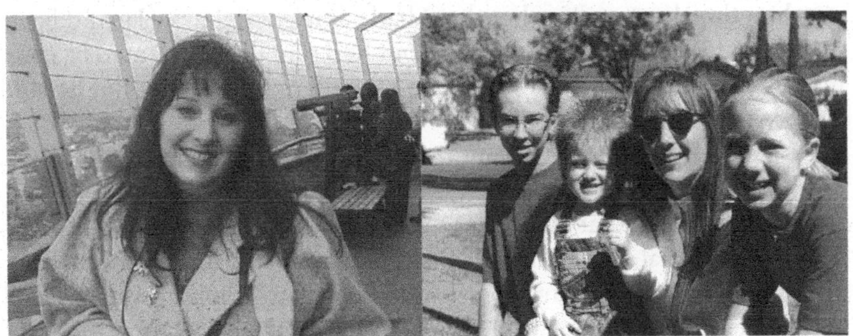

by Debbie Martin

In 1999, I found out that I was pregnant with baby number four. I already had three children in sixteen years with my first husband – who was verbally and emotionally (and occasionally, physically) abusive.

In 1996, I met the man of my dreams. He'd shown me unconditional love, and he loved my children just as much as he loved me. We'd only had one fight in almost three years, and our second fight had just started.

We were actors who met when we were cast as lovers in a musical. We fell so much in love, so quickly, and soon we were spending every moment possible together. Just eight months after we met, we moved in together. The biggest problem we had was my jealousy over him having to kiss his leading ladies in the musicals where he was mostly cast as the leading man.

I was a young, very insecure woman, thus the second fight. I was terribly threatened by the young woman cast opposite him in the latest musical in which he'd started rehearsals.

At that time, I had started having some abdominal pain and an irregular period, so I went to see my doctor. He did an ultrasound and some blood work, sending me home with a promise to call me later that afternoon.

That night, my soon-to-be-husband had rehearsal. Before supper, I voiced, yet again, my unhappiness that he'd be kissing the actress playing his girlfriend in the show. He got mad and left. I knew he'd gone to his sister's house; that's where he always went when he was upset about something.

Those were the days before caller ID and cell phones, so when the phone rang, I hoped it was him, calling to tell me how much he loved me and that he'd see me later that night after rehearsal. Instead, it was my doctor, telling me the happiest news. I was pregnant! (I had been on birth control so it was an incredible surprise.) I was overjoyed! I immediately called my future sister-in-law and asked if my fiancé was there. She hesitantly told me that he was, and I asked to speak to him. I was crushed when she told me that he wouldn't take my call. I begged her to give him the phone, telling her that I had some good news. (He did have one daughter from his first marriage, but he'd said that he wanted to have more children, so I knew he would be happy with this news.) But he still wouldn't take my call.

I was so upset that after I put the kids to bed, I cried and cried. I anguished over my insecurities and his rejection of me. I wasn't even sure he would come home that night after rehearsal, and I cried even harder.

I waited up late, and when he finally walked in the door, I flew into his arms, unwilling to fight anymore. I immediately told him my good news, and just as I had hoped he would be, he was overjoyed. This time, the tears were of relief and joy.

All I could think about was how excited we both were about having a baby. This was our child. His and mine. I calculated the due date, and fantasized about how we would tell the children. I was SURE this baby was a sweet little girl.

You know how it is when you find out that you're pregnant – you're instantly in love with the new little life growing inside you. It doesn't matter if you've just found out you're pregnant, or if you've known for months. The love makes your heart swell as that little life wraps your heart around its little finger.

Just two days later, I instinctively knew something was wrong. My doctor had me come in, this time for a vaginal ultrasound, and he confirmed my worst fear – I was having a miscarriage. I was devastated, but at the same time, I wouldn't believe it! I somehow hoped and believed that he was wrong (even though he was the best doctor in our area), but the blood that kept coming told me that he was right. Our dream of holding that precious baby girl in our arms would never come true. Instead, the dream had turned into a nightmare. We were crushed.

As I write this, my sweet baby girl would be nearing twenty-one years old. Time has flown; it seems like it's been just a few short years.

It's only been in the last couple of years that I can think of her without crying. Knowing that I'm really a mama of four sweet babies, not just the three live ones (that are now adults) can be bittersweet. My other children don't even know that they'd almost had a baby sister. I've only told a handful of people about her, until now.

Over the years, I've felt like I needed to keep her existence to myself. I thought that because I'd only been pregnant such a short time, that I shouldn't be so upset about losing her. And I blamed myself for the miscarriage. If only I hadn't been so jealous. If only I hadn't been so upset about him kissing someone else. If only I hadn't cried so hard, maybe she'd be alive today.

As I write this, I shake my head at the crazy things grief does to us. Now that I'm older (and feel like I've lived a couple of lifetimes), and have talked to other women who have also blamed themselves for their miscarriages, I realize that it wasn't my fault.

I wonder what she would have looked like. Would she have had her daddy's jet-black hair, or her mama's green eyes? Would she be a singer like the both of us? Would she be as passionate about theatre and entertaining as her daddy and me? Would she adore her daddy and be her mama's best friend? I'll never know. But I think she's been my guardian angel, especially these last seven years, as I've fought to make a life for and by myself after her daddy decided to forge a different path in life with someone else, further breaking my heart and devastating me.

One day, I'll be in Heaven and get to meet my little Angel. I don't know what Heaven will be like, but I like to imagine that we will get to know each other over tea and luscious desserts; and that I'll be able to tell her about her sisters and brothers and we'll never be separated again.

Public Figures Share Their Personal Experiences To Help Others

Mary Tyler Moore – *6 weeks. Unknown/Undisclosed.*

"As we were preparing to do the series, a surprise pregnancy gave the promise of a huge event. So, Grant and I set about the fun of telling anyone who'd listen that we were embarking on a production of another sort. In about six weeks' time the promise was broken. This growing expression of us both ended in its beginning. And the loss took my heart with it as well."

From her book *Growing Up Again: Life, Loves, and Oh Yeah, Diabetes,* published in 2009.

2

Pip's Story

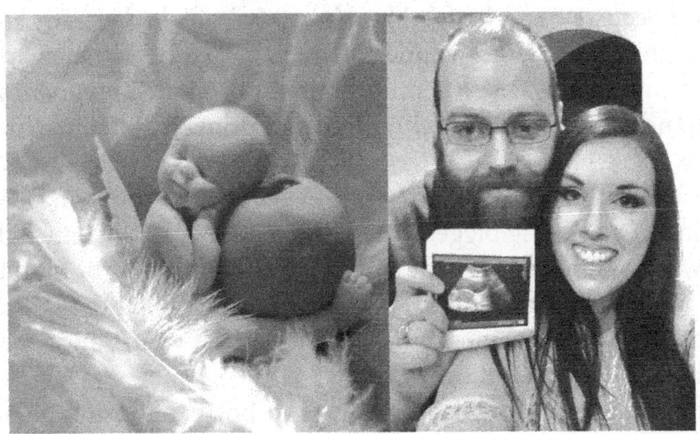

by Rose Skillcorn

I have wanted my own family for as long as I can remember. Even as a child, all my games and imagining revolved around having a family; a child to love, a baby to nurse, mums and dads; lulling my dolls to sleep. Knowing this, you can imagine the worry when my husband and I discovered that having a baby wasn't going to be as straight-forward as it was for most people. My heart felt crushed, but my need to be a mother was far too strong and engrained in me to let it stop me. It is the beat of my heart.

We went through the invasive procedures, (the vaginal examinations, the semen analysis, running dye through my fallopian tubes etc.) and the trials and tribulations of running all my womanly functions through the hospital. I had an operation to remove a cyst in one of my fallopian tubes and took the pills the doctor gave me, but nothing worked and we were told I had polycystic ovarian syndrome and unexplained infertility. Our best chance was IVF.

It was then that I learned IVF wasn't an easy fix. There was injection after injection. It's not a fear of mine, but I have been through menopause six times already through IVF and I am only 30. My first round was unsuccessful and on the second round, my body didn't respond to the medication. After two years, I finally got pregnant with my little miracle. I had dreamed and dreamed of the day I could finally look at my husband and say, "I'm pregnant!" I had imagined that moment in my head, over and over again, and when the day came that it was true, the magical moment transcended all my hopes and dreams. It felt better than I have ever imagined.

We nicknamed him Pip, because when he was the size of an apple seed, it just kind of stuck. I was absolutely confident Pip was a boy; there wasn't one tiny thought in my mind that made me think of the possibility of a girl, because to me, he felt like a boy. My body had already started to change in mysterious and wonderful ways. I was already having morning sickness, though it was pretty mild, (but it was my first pregnancy and so in my mind, it was horrendous). I look back now and realize how tough it can be.

I was just about to nip into work to get a larger uniform, seeing as I was going to be getting bigger, when I noticed that I had some light spotting. I was five weeks pregnant and it was the tiniest bit of blood. It was hardly anything but I went into full panic mode, calling the IVF clinic in an absolutely hysterical mess. They told me that it wasn't uncommon and to up the IVF medication I was taking.

When you go through IVF, you have both suppositories and oral medication to take. These support the pregnancy until you are twelve weeks along and your body is producing the hormones itself. So, I did as I was told; I upped the medication and hoped for the best. My Mum, who had gone through five miscarriages in her life, told me I needed to take it really easy. So, the next day, I didn't really do anything. I put my feet up and snuggled closely with my kitty cat. There hadn't been any more blood and I was feeling relieved. Surely, it was just a tiny blip in my beautiful journey with a happy ending.

It was that evening, before my husband was home from work, that I realized it wasn't just a blip. I sat watching a movie and when it finished, I realized I had been constantly rocking backwards and forwards, subconsciously, because of a pain in my tummy. I ran to the toilet and was greeted with bright red blood. My head spun, my heart lurched, I was full of panic. *How could this be happening? This can't be happening! It can't! This was my miracle!* I told my husband immediately when he got home and he took me straight to the clinic.

Luckily the clinic was still open and they scanned me there and then. In my tummy was my beautiful little Pip, and his heart was beating! I cannot quite describe the relief that flooded me when I saw his little body, not yet even resembling a baby, but healthy and happy. It put my heart at ease. I felt so confident that my little apple Pip was going to be fine. He was a fighter, just like his Mum, who had fought through years of infertility. But the nightmare didn't end there.

The next couple of weeks were a blur. My mum would come 'round and do some jobs for me. I remained on strict bed rest, only moving to go to the toilet. It was Operation Keeping Pip. I was told again and again by my family, friends, and even the IVF nurses, that I must stay positive for the baby. I was told it was so, so common in an IVF pregnancy to bleed, sometimes all the way through the pregnancy. So, there I was, sending my beautiful little Pip positive energy, and redirecting my attention if my head started to race with the "What ifs?" and negative thinking. Every single time my thoughts would stray, I would nudge them right back to love and peace and calm. I told Pip how much I loved him, to hold on and keep fighting. I knew he couldn't hear me because he wasn't developed enough yet, but I was a great believer in energy, and knew if I was comforted and calm, he would be too.

I was back and forth to the hospital, in immense pain, for tests, Beta tests, comparison tests. On paper, I was pregnant and my sweet boy was holding on. But inside, my uterus griped and large clots squeezed through my closed cervix. I was put on the early assessment ward and given morphine and gas and air. I was in there for six hours. The nurses couldn't really tell me anything. They just kept repeating, "When you are bleeding and passing clots when pregnant, it is cause for concern." NO! I wouldn't believe it. I was not going to admit defeat. Pip was my boy, a miracle I had worked for, for three whole years of my life. In my head, the persistent encouraging words of my family and the IVF clinic whizzed round. *BE POSITIVE!* Me and my boy were going to beat this. I went home. The hospital couldn't offer me anything other than pain medication.

That night when I got into bed, there came an intense, searing pain in my womb. I felt sick, hot, and shaky. I squeezed my mouth shut to keep from screaming. I tried to stay calm and went to the bathroom without alerting my husband that anything was different. When I got to the bathroom the biggest clot yet came out. I looked at it for a long time. That was him. Wasn't it? That had to be him. I told my husband, but we had been told to remain positive. We put it down to another clot. We had to stay positive. That was at six and a half weeks.

At seven weeks I had a scan. My Pip was gone! My heart shattered into smithereens. I had fought so hard for him but I hadn't done enough. He was gone. My husband and I sobbed. We were taken to IVF, where all the happy people becoming pregnant were; where our life had just dropped out from under us. I stayed angry at God for the longest time. Why was it, that someone so ready for a baby was so unlucky? The hospital kept calling it an early miscarriage – like that made a difference. My boy was real; his heart was beating.

Eventually, for some peace, we named him Pip-Mason (after I had a dream about him and that name kept sticking in my head). But I battled every day, watching my friends and family get pregnant around me. I was broken when I saw big bumps and glowing mothers, broken when the next pregnancy announcement came along, broken when I opened my curtains on a morning and saw the school run. I would cry in the shower and wail around the house; just walking, my inside slightly fractured. Eventually, two years later, I got pregnant again through IVF. I was over the moon, beyond happy. I promised myself I would tell our baby of her strong and sweet brother in heaven. I gave birth to my sweet Liliana Grace. She died after 15 fifteen days spent in the NICU, bravely fighting with an amazing courage. She is my Warrior Princess. My heart remains broken. I am right in the middle of deep, debilitating sorrow. My only comfort is that Pip and Liliana are together in heaven. A few days after we buried Liliana, a little baby was buried opposite her; his name was Mason. This brought me great comfort, to know that they were in each other's company, a synchronicity, like it was spoken from heaven.

Seven months after my latest loss I write this, still with the deepest ache in my heart and overcome with unimaginable grief. I write poems and songs of my two angels in heaven. They lift my music to a deeper place. I sing of them often and honor them, Pip on his due date (15 November) and Liliana on her birthday (29 November). My Autumn stars. I will love them forever and long to hold them until the day I will meet them again.

Public Figures Share Their Personal Experiences To Help Others

Lisa Ling – *7 weeks. Missed miscarriage.*

"I felt more like a failure than I'd felt in a very long time.

"We actually [hadn't] been trying that long. I don't know that I took it as seriously as I should have because it happened so fast. But then when I heard the doctor say there was no heartbeat it was like bam, like a knife through the heart."

https://people.com/celebrity/lisa-ling-i-had-a-miscarriage/

Young Love

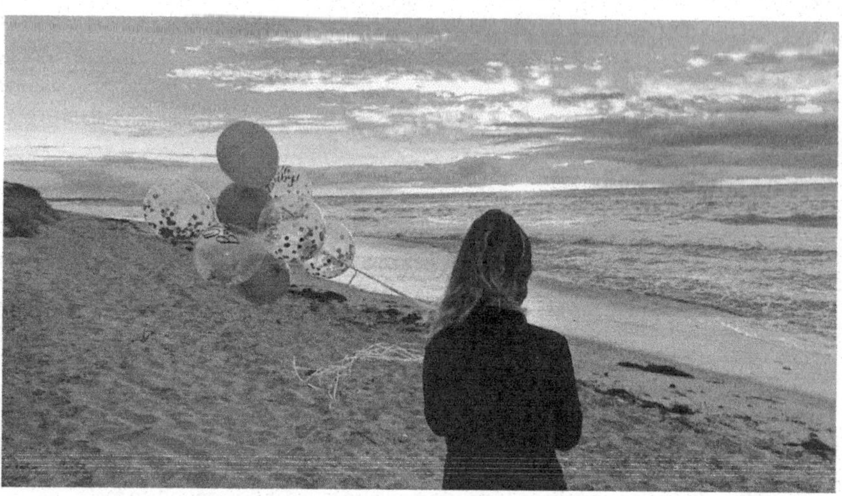

by Luci Sorgiovanni

Since I was a little girl, I have always dreamed about being a mummy. I grew up in a family of eight and have always been surrounded by babies and young kids. Never did I think I would fall pregnant at sixteen. My boyfriend and I basically ignored the fact that I was pregnant and never really spoke about it, as he was a very anxious person.

I found out when I was roughly seven weeks along. I was sick and had cravings of chocolate cake and Sour Patch Kids. To this day, I can't eat either without feeling empty and upset. I miscarried during Covid-19, so I was self-isolating with my family and not seeing my boyfriend, which was already hard as I was used to seeing him at least five times a week, if not more. On the night all of this went down, which was the 7th of April, I was in my room. I had not been feeling the best all day, then I started bleeding. I thought to myself that it was just "implantation" bleeding and everything was fine. It wasn't that but I was in denial; the bleeding got worse and so did the cramps and back pain.

I told my boyfriend on the phone while crying. His step-mother is a nurse, so he told her and asked her for advice. She said it sounded like I might be having a miscarriage. That night, I sat on the floor of the shower crying my eyes out. By the time I got out, the blood seemed as if it had gotten worse. I sat on my bedroom floor, naked, on a towel that was catching my baby, now just clots and blood.

Unfortunately, I now suffer from PTSD and depression, and I am still getting help for that to this day. What happened on the 7th of April will always be one of the most traumatic experiences of my life. I found this time very difficult as I felt alone in my grief.

I ended up joining a few miscarriage groups on Facebook to see if there was anyone else as young as me. I read through hundreds of posts and sadly, didn't seem to find anyone around the same age. I was extremely nervous the first time I posted in the groups as I didn't know what sort of comments I would get, being so young. I got nothing but support from these women. I was thrilled with this and didn't feel so alone.

I will forever think about the what-ifs. I would be 26 weeks today, but sadly, my baby is now my angel. Since my miscarriage, I refer to my angel as, "My Rainbow." When my boyfriend and I see rainbows we both think of our baby.

To the ladies that are going through a miscarriage: you are not alone.

Public Figures Share Their Personal Experiences To Help Others

Nancy Kerrigan – *Multiple miscarriages. Unknown/Undisclosed.*

I always thought I'd have three kids by the time I was 30.

The first time that you go in and they tell you, "Oh there's no heartbeat," it's devastating. I felt like a failure.

Once the pregnancy was far enough along that we actually told our son and he was so excited ... How do you explain [a miscarriage] to a little kid? Having to tell them that it was now gone and they had to take it out? He asked why and we had to explain, "Because it's dead. It's not alive anymore." That was awful.

Jerry asked me if I was sure I wanted to keep going. It was hard for him to see me hurting. But I wasn't ready to stop trying.

I think about it now and remember we couldn't come up with a name for Brian. I wonder if we probably were afraid to come up with a name because that makes you close and we could lose him.

[In trying for a final child] there were two eggs left and they said, "Do you want both?" And we were, like, "Oh." Sometimes people get twins and that would have been okay before Brian, but we already had two now so we said no. They said, 'This one looks strong!' But then it wasn't strong and they said it didn't work. Then they said "There's only this weak one left," which is funny because our daughter Nicole is the complete opposite of weak.... Now we're outnumbered.

https://people.com/celebrity/dwts-nancy-kerrigan-devastating-miscarriages-exclusive-video/

4

WAITING ON A RAINBOW

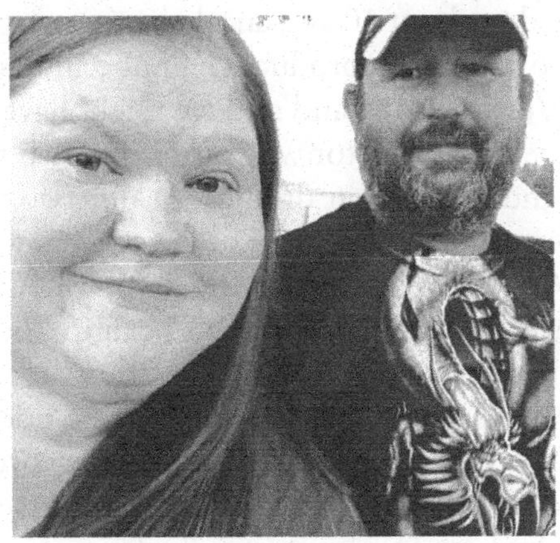

by Jessica Oberlin

I started dating the man of my dreams in 2005. During that time, I stopped having periods consistently. I went to a local OBGYN who said, "You have Polycystic Ovarian Syndrome (PCOS); if you want children, you might as well give up that dream. You're overweight, and with PCOS, it will just never happen." At 18 years old, I was young, carefree, and just thought, *Oh well, I'll adopt.*

Then, on September 10th, 2011, we got married. We decided we wanted a second opinion. This time, the doctor said, "You're young; we will get you pregnant no problem!" And they did! After the third cycle with Clomid, and timed intercourse, we were pregnant. At what would have been 8 weeks pregnant, we discovered that my hCG only got to 300, then it had drastically dropped and we would have a miscarriage. We were heartbroken but told, "These things happen; chromosomes come together quickly and sometimes there's just issues."

We tried for another 3 three years with no luck. Then, on my 27th birthday, we did our second round of Clomid and IUI, and we got pregnant! We were so excited; surely, we wouldn't have another chromosome issue, but sadly, I miscarried again. This time, the hCG never went past 150. And again, "These things happen; chromosomes come together quickly, but you're young." We then decided to go to a fertility specialist.

Our first meeting with the fertility specialist was a positive one; they found possible polyps in my uterus and the doctor was sure that was the cause of my miscarriages, since my OBGYN had run RPL bloodwork and everything was normal. We had surgery and after our second round of IUI and medication, we were pregnant again. The day after the positive beta test, I began spotting. The doctor said it was normal. Our next beta didn't quite double but it was pretty close. Our beta was 50; by the next beta, it had dropped to about 10 and another miscarriage happened.

We changed to another reproductive endocrinologist who suggested a hysteroscopy/laparoscopy and said we might have an auto-immune issue. I had surgery by this doctor who also suggested they open my left tube, if possible, and do ovarian drilling. At our two-week post-op appointment, we were told we could try to get pregnant again. We started the medication. We were pregnant on the first try. Our betas were doubling like they never had before. We got a beautiful heartbeat from our miracle, then, at six weeks, I was diagnosed with a subchorionic hematoma, and at seven weeks, we found out our baby did not have a heartbeat. Another miscarriage. We were able to try again after two cycles. We tried for a total of four cycles of medicated, timed intercourse but they were all negative. We were bummed and emotionally drained and decided to take a break. A few months later, I wasn't feeling right and I took a pregnancy test; the second line came right up right away. We couldn't believe it; we were pregnant on our own with no medication. The next day, I went for blood work and an ultrasound. My beta was almost 30,000; we were so excited. Then we went for our ultrasound and heard, "I'm sorry but your baby does not have a heartbeat." We were so devastated.

Why does this keep happening? What did we do wrong? What did we do to deserve this? All of these questions play through my head a lot. I try to remind myself that our babies only knew love and that brings me a lot of comfort. I also have to remember that we did nothing wrong! We didn't cause this! We also have bought a little angel for each loss and framed the ultrasound pictures of our fourth and fifth losses. I often think of our babies and wonder who they would have been. What would they have liked? What wouldn't they have liked? Would they have looked like me or their dad? While the rest of the world may never understand our pain, we do! Don't let people downplay or disregard your grief. Our babies matter and were wanted and loved.We are ready to try again because for us, the thought of not being parents is harder than the thought of having another angel. Our faith and our love for one another has brought us this far and I couldn't imagine going through this with anyone else.

If I could give advice to myself, I would say, "Be kind to yourself; this isn't your fault. If you feel something is wrong, follow your gut; don't stay with the same doctors that aren't changing your treatment plan when you have multiple losses. Allow yourself to grieve and separate emotionally from those that try to disregard your pain. Everyone grieves in their own way; just because it's not the same as yours, doesn't mean your loss doesn't matter to them. Reach out and get help when the depression kicks in, don't wait. And again, be kind to yourself!"

We are ready to try again.

5

Joy in the Mourning

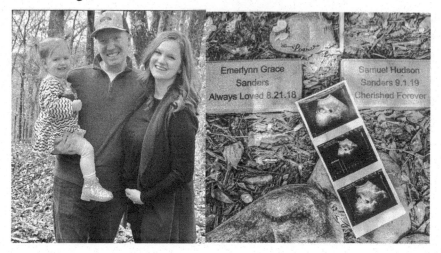

by Tabitha Saunders

"I can't find a heartbeat." These five words still replay in my mind two and a half years later. My husband and I were eight weeks and one day pregnant when we were told our first baby had stopped growing ten days prior and did not have a heartbeat. My doctor remained hopeful and requested we come back the following week because he suspected I miscalculated how far along I could be and hoped that was why the heartbeat could not be detected. I left the appointment with a knot in my stomach because I knew miscalculation was not an option; I knew my baby was gone.

If you knew me, you would know I am a perfectionist. I had been meticulously calculating all of the details of when I would be ovulating for almost a year in an attempt to get pregnant. When we finally had a positive pregnancy test, I was naïve to the thought that we could miscarry. We quickly had announcement pictures taken and announced our pregnancy on Christmas. After the miscarriage, I learned that news of our pregnancy had spread. People that I did not know came up to me in the store congratulating me on our pregnancy, not knowing that we had lost our baby.

Guilt, fear, depression, and anger surrounded me. I felt guilty that I could not carry our baby for my husband. I was afraid we would not conceive again. I felt angry that women around me were having babies, and I was not. Depression seeped in as holidays and my lost little girl's due date approached.

Eleven months later, on Christmas Eve, I had another positive pregnancy test. For the second Christmas in a row, my husband and I were celebrating a pregnancy. The excitement of a rainbow baby quickly faded into sadness as I lost him the day after Christmas. After multiple blood tests and an appointment where I sat across from my sweet doctor, repeatedly asking, "Why?" I learned we'd had a chemical pregnancy.

My husband and I proudly tell people we are parents of three children – one on Earth and two in Heaven. We named our babies and had pavers placed at the National Memorial for the Unborn in Chattanooga, Tennessee. We bring our new baby to visit her siblings, and we decorate the pavers for every holiday. I find comfort in visiting Emerlynn and Samuel when sadness, fear, and guilt find their way back in.

We never felt more alone or more pain than the months after we lost our babies. We are learning that we are not alone and that there is a tribe of men and women that are also walking this path of healing. We tell our story because hearing the stories of others helped us. Miscarriage and chemical pregnancies are such taboo topics, but they are a part of so many of our stories. Grieving and healing from these losses is a journey, a journey I will always be on. It made me who I am. It made me a mom.

Public Figures Share Their Personal Experiences To Help Others

Elisabetta Canalis – *Miscarriage. Unknown/Undisclosed.*

Unfortunately, life gives you ... a reality that you do not expect. That is very hard to accept, even if you think you are strong.

You're never really ready to be told that there is no more beating (heartbeat) and that it had already stopped long ago.

I just want to say to all those women who are going through it to stay strong. Life goes on and it is nobody's fault and nature acts in incomprehensible ways.

We can only accept it. I just want to say that I feel you close, if you are suffering as I am doing. We can't deny it, it's like an incessant sorrow you can't get rid of.

post on WhoSay https://www.her.ie/celeb/elisabetta-canalis-speaks-out-about-miscarriage-148253

7

Broken to Blessed

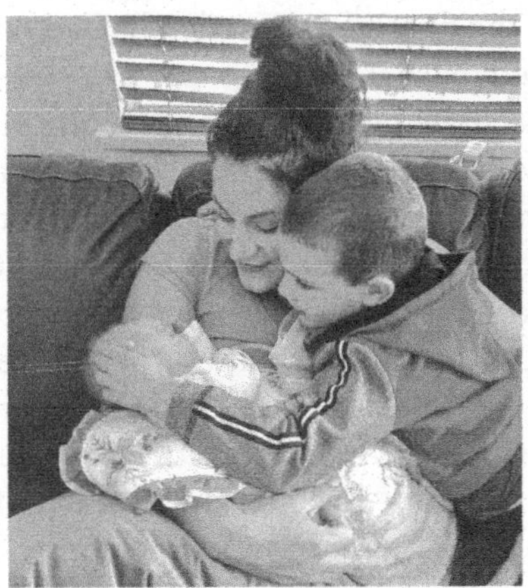

by Kayla Jones

I never thought it would happen to me. Why would it? My first-born son was textbook. Everything went as it should and I gave birth to a beautiful healthy boy. For as long as I can remember, all I wanted was to get married, have kids, and raise all of them with the huge amount of love I had in my heart.

I pictured my life working out a certain way, on a certain timeline. So, after having my son in 2015, my husband and I decided to wait so that there would be two to three years between our children, as per my original plan. In 2017, we had just moved into a new home, had amazing jobs, were financially sound, and had a happy, healthy toddler. It was time. We began trying for our second child.

After six months of no such luck, it was finally there: the second pink line. We had conceived on my birthday and I tested four days early, riddled with hope and anxiety. About seven weeks into my pregnancy, I was at work and started feeling some intense lower abdominal pain, which I thought could have been related to the GI issues I have had off and on, but considering my pregnancy, I wanted to be safe. I drove myself to the nearest walk-in clinic and was assessed by a lovely doctor. She tested my urine for HCG and told me I needed to go to emergency immediately, as the line on my pregnancy test was more faint than it should be at seven weeks; she worried it was an ectopic pregnancy. I burst into tears, called my husband in a panic, and then my best friend (who was closer to me in location) for a ride to the ER.

After waiting for what felt like an eternity to hear the results of my ultrasound and blood-work, the ER doctor came waltzing in to my room and excitedly stated, "I have great news! It's not an ectopic pregnancy ... However, I don't believe it is viable." Those words hit me like a ton of bricks. How could this possibly be "great news?" My eyes welled with tears. Only then did the doctor realize what he had said and try to make it better. Nothing would make it better.

After three weeks of living in limbo and having blood work and ultrasounds regularly, a very kind and warm OB finally made the call and told me our little bean would not grow, and sadly, would not make it. I had to make the decision to wait and let it pass naturally (all while having my placenta continue to grow, and continuing to *feel* pregnant for however long it would take), or to have a D and C, at ten weeks. I couldn't bear the thought of carrying this dead child inside me with no hope. I opted to have a D and C, which was booked on the exact date my son was born three years prior, in the same hospital, and same unit. It was devastating and surreal. I awoke from the surgery feeling empty, both physically and emotionally. My uterus was empty and my heart was broken.

After some time to grieve, collect the pieces of our broken hearts, and regain some hope, we decided to start trying again. This time, I was anxious, nervous, and sometimes terrified. I kept telling myself, *The chances of two consecutive miscarriages are so slim, it's bound to work out this time.* Six anxiety-riddled months later, I was pregnant again! But this time, it felt different. I was less hopeful, more anxious, and scared. Something inside was not allowing me to feel excited or happy. Something felt wrong, but still, I told myself, *Statistics are in our favor*. Nine weeks into this pregnancy, we lost our little one again. This time, I started bleeding; as soon as I saw the blood, I knew. My mother and best friend told me not to worry, that spotting was normal. But I knew. The next day, I made another trip to the ER where it was confirmed: there was no hope. Every part of me felt broken and confused.

Why? Does God not want me to raise another child? Does he not want my son to have a sibling? Am I being punished for the sins of my past? Maybe the universe is trying to tell me something. Maybe I should just give up. Once again, we collected the pieces of our broken hearts, pulled ourselves together, and focused on trying to figure out why. That was the question I so desperately needed answered. I was referred to a fertility specialist and went through every blood test, ultrasound, imaging, and procedure in order to try and figure it out. But everything was normal. There was nothing obvious that could have caused this to happen twice in a row. So, I suppose it was the luck of the draw? Or as the fertility doctor told me, "The universe's way of sparing you a much worse fate."

No one understood; everyone kept telling me to stay strong and keep trying, that it would work out eventually. Others said, "At least it was early," or, "Could you imagine if it happened later in the pregnancy?" As if my loss was not as big simply because my babies were younger and underdeveloped. My own mother brushed it off as if I shouldn't feel so much sadness. My father kept asking what was wrong with me for this to happen. I felt guilty and ashamed. I shut down. I stopped talking to people and decided to carry on silently. I couldn't handle my losses being compared to others'. I started to feel like I didn't have a right to feel sadness, to feel broken and empty; that I should be grateful I had one healthy son. I didn't think I would have another child.

After two courses of a fertility medication prescribed by the doctor, I was once again pregnant after a few months of trying. This time I held my breath. I told no one. I waited, seven weeks ... eight weeks ... nine weeks ... and then, before I knew it, I was twelve weeks along. The anxiety started to settle and for the first time in a while, I believed I was going to have another baby. Every day of that pregnancy, I worried. I feared the worst. I was drowning in anxiety but trying desperately to keep calm in order to have a healthy pregnancy.

I am so very happy to say that I gave birth to a beautiful, healthy baby girl. My son has a sibling, and I have the most precious gift I could ever ask for. The birth of my daughter filled the emptiness I felt for the three years we tried to make her. But I am still left wondering who the other two would have been, and a part of me feels guilty for being happy and for loving my daughter beyond measure. I believe I will always feel this way.

Loss is loss, no matter how and when it occurs. It may hurt differently with different situations, but it hurts nonetheless. All I can say is that I am blessed, I am grateful, and I will never take either of my children for granted. I will always feel love and sadness for the two that didn't make it, but I truly believe that God had a different plan for them, and for me.

Public Figures Share Their Personal Experiences To Help Others

Sofia Loren – *Miscarriage. Low estrogen*

"By the time I reached the age of 29, my desire to have children had become an obsession. I simply loved children. On the sets of my movies, I'd befriend the child actors and then stay in touch with them long after shooting had finished.

"Recently, the little girl who acted with me in Houseboat in 1957 wrote to say she'd just become a grandmother.

"But in 1963 — when 29 was considered old to be a first-time mother — I was wondering if it would ever happen.

"Coincidentally, I started getting what seemed like pregnancy symptoms while playing a mother-of-seven in a film being shot in Naples.

"For a few days, I put them down to the fact I was playing a mother and identifying so much with my role.

"But finally I went to a doctor, who did some tests — and they came back negative. "However, my strange feeling wouldn't go away. Next, a supposed expert from Rome arrived, carrying a dark leather briefcase. When he opened it, I jumped: it contained a tiny green frog which was staring at me, his eyes bulging with fright.

To my horror, the doctor injected it with some of my urine, saying: 'If the frog dies, it means you're pregnant . . .'

"It wasn't long before the frog started moving around erratically, as if it had been hit on the head. But it didn't die. Disgusted, I got rid of the doctor and went out for a walk, releasing the poor creature into a pond.

"'Too bad,' I said to myself. 'For a moment there, I thought I was pregnant.' Incredibly, I was. I was desperately happy, happier than I'd ever been before, and couldn't wait to look my own child in the eyes. But that's not how it turned out. The following days were among the saddest and darkest of my life. I could tell something wasn't right.

"I went to see another doctor, who reassured me but told me not to travel by car so I headed to Milan, the movie's next location, by train.

"Unfortunately, my first scene took place almost entirely in a stage car mounted on a hydraulic arm to simulate the bumps. It was much worse than any real car.

"That first night in Milan, I felt a terrible pain. As I got into the hotel lift, I almost fainted. I can still see myself lying on that hospital bed, under strip lighting, surrounded by white walls, and with the smell of disinfectant penetrating my every cell and piercing my heart.

"My most painful recollection of that night was the scornful look on the faces of the nurses — who were nuns. They all seemed to blame me.

"Like the rest of the world, they knew that I wasn't married to my partner, the film producer Carlo Ponti. (His first marriage had broken up years before but divorce was still illegal in Italy.)

"Of course, those nuns thought they knew the real story, but they didn't know anything about me, my desires and my fears. They were insensitive, inhumane, devoid of feeling. Their gratuitous humiliation of me was spurred by prejudice and ignorance.

I lost the baby.

"Afterwards, I went straight back to work. But I felt gutted. It was as if the world had been turned off for ever. I could see nothing to look forward to, nothing that could ever console me.

"My life as a star felt like nothing compared with the happiness of the new mothers I'd glimpsed at the hospital, getting ready to breastfeed their newborn babies.

"Four years later, I got pregnant again while making *More Than A Miracle.*

"I was more prepared: at the first signs, I called Carlo to say: 'I'm pregnant. But this time I'm going to be careful; I don't want to take any risks.' I forced myself to stay in bed. I did nothing: I didn't read, didn't watch TV, I even spoke as little as possible and avoided touching my stomach in case it bothered the baby.

"But a little voice inside was telling me that the same thing was happening all over again.

At the first signs of the pain that I remembered all too well, I was at home with my dear friend Basilio at our beautiful villa in the Roman hills, while Carlo was in London for work. It was Basilio who called the doctor: 'Come quickly, please. She's having contractions, she's as white as a ghost and she feels faint.'

"But my great and mighty doctor said with arrogant self-confidence: 'It's nothing to worry about. Have her drink some chamomile; we'll talk about it tomorrow.'

"Despite this, we rushed to the hospital — and happened to run into the doctor, who was about to leave for a cocktail party.

Before leaving, he gave me a strong sedative.

"'It's just a passing crisis,' he declared, his white coat fluttering over his cashmere sweater. 'Now, try to get some sleep.'

"The contractions were getting worse, as if I were in labour, and my face was as yellow as a lemon. At this, my mother — who'd just joined us — pounced on him with all her strength. 'Can't you see her face? She's having a miscarriage!' she cried.

"But nothing doing. The great man's cocktail party couldn't wait.

"When my pains suddenly stopped at 4am, I knew it was all over. The doctor was called but took two hours to get to the hospital. 'Signora,' he told me, 'you no doubt have excellent hips, and you're a beautiful woman, but you will never have a child.'

"His scathing words dashed all my hopes, making me feel powerless, barren and deeply inadequate.

"'Now I can go back to the set and finish the movie,' I said to Carlo as soon as he arrived. I was trying to lighten the blow, to show him how strong I was.

"His smile turned into a grimace; it was obvious that he felt totally helpless. Only at that moment did I let myself go, crying my heart out.

"In the desperate months that followed, a sense of failure spread to every corner of my soul. Even Carlo — a solid, concrete businessman — became depressed. He could hardly work, talk or smile.

"Luckily, fate led us to an unexpected discovery. The wife of an Italian film director had gone through an odyssey similar to mine, but she'd chanced upon an internationally renowned expert who'd helped her carry to term.

"His name was Hubert de Watteville, and he was the director of the gynaecology clinic at Geneva Hospital in Switzerland.

"Tall and very thin, de Watteville was about 60, with a beaklike nose and a somewhat aristocratic, detached air.

"My heart sank: I'd hoped he'd be more of a sympathetic father-figure.

"But I was mistaken in my first impression. He hadn't had any children himself, and he'd poured his desire for fatherhood into his work, so that the children he helped come into the world were in some ways his.

"After studying my case, he told me: 'There's nothing wrong — you're a very normal woman. The next time you get pregnant, we'll monitor you closely.'

So, in early 1968, when I got pregnant for the third time, I moved to Geneva. I chose a hotel close to the doctor's office, took to my bed and waited patiently for him to perform a miracle

"He concluded that my body wasn't producing enough oestrogen, which was stopping the egg from attaching to the uterus. This, however, was easily solved with oestrogen injections.

"Meanwhile, I had months of forced idleness on the 18th floor of the Hotel Intercontinental.

"To distract myself, I spent hours recreating the recipes from my Naples childhood — and years later, published them as a cookbook. Finally the day came when I was due to have a C-section. I hadn't slept a wink the night before; the truth is that I didn't want my pregnancy to end.

"And I was scared. I didn't want to share this child that was all mine with anyone else. A few hours later, Carlo Jr. was born — the greatest, sweetest, most indescribable joy I had ever experienced. I was completely overcome by emotion when I held him in my arms."

https://www.dailymail.co.uk/femail/article-2810225/Losing-two-babies-feel-failure-woman-Sophia-Loren-reveals-suffered-heart-break-two-miscarriages-fulfilling-dream-mother-last.html

7

Why, God?

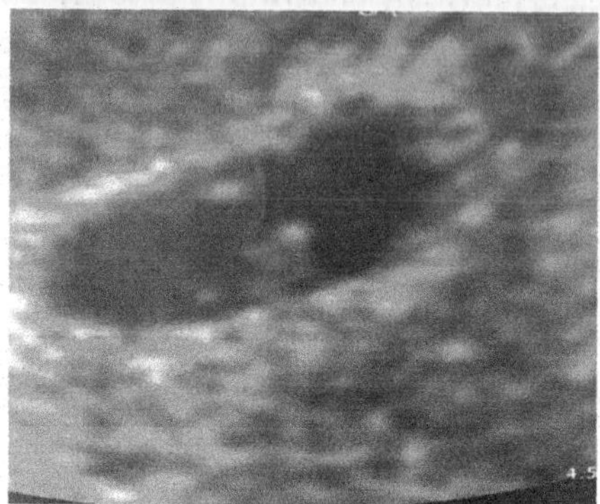

by Amanda Wong Loi Sing

I remember seeing that positive pregnancy test and freaking out. *We already have three kids under four, how am I going to handle another?* That quickly turned to excitement but then I started to bleed, not a lot but enough to be concerning. I went into my OBGYN's office and an ultrasound was performed. Nothing could be found that was wrong; I just wasn't as far along as we had thought. The bleeding continued off and on but then we finally saw a little baby and a heartbeat. I thought I was in the clear, but a couple of weeks later, the baby had not grown. I was still bleeding and my gestational sac was shrinking. There was a heartbeat but I was told it was inevitable that I was going to lose the baby.

That baby's heartbeat hung on until the day before I miscarried. It took about two weeks and the heartache was the worst thing I had ever felt. My baby was alive but would inevitably die. I had to deal with that pain for two weeks. I begged God to take it and get it over with. I was drowning in my sorrows. I began to feel abandoned by God. *How could a loving God let me go through something so cruel?* I cried a lot in those two weeks and struggled to care for my other children. My oldest, who is four, just couldn't stand to see me sad and it broke my heart even more that it was affecting her too, but the grief was so deep, I was lost in it. Then, on Christmas Eve, 2019, when I should have been about nine weeks pregnant, I started bleeding profusely and was rushed to the E.R. where I had to endure more heartache because E.R. doctors really don't get it when it comes to miscarriages.

I lay there on the bed for a couple hours, bleeding, passing clots, not knowing if my baby was in there somewhere or not, and then my blood pressure dropped. The OBGYN on call was finally brought in and I was given a D&C. I felt a lot better after that but it was short lived as the hormonal and mental crap set in, along with needing a blood transfusion.

I struggled for a few months to regain a grip on my mental health. I journaled a lot and sought out a counselor (who has been an absolute godsend) and slowly, I've pulled out of it. I can say I'm in a pretty good place right now. I don't know why this happened to me, but I have faith I will see that baby one day and faith in the plan that God has for all of it, whatever that may be. It's so hard to trust in God's promises, especially during such a hard time, but he is God and as hard as it is, I have to trust Him.

Public Figures Share Their Personal Experiences To Help Others

Pink – *Multiple miscarriages. Unknown /Undisclosed.*

"Since I was 17, I've always hated my body and it feels like my body's hated me".

"I've always had this very tomboy, very strong gymnast body, but actually at 17 I had a miscarriage ... I was going to have that child. But when that happens to a woman or a young girl, you feel like your body hates you and like your body is broken, and it's not doing what it's supposed to do. I've had several miscarriages since so I think it's important to talk about what you're ashamed of, who you really are and the painful shit. I've always written that way. I believe in self-confrontation and just getting things out."

Not only did Pink use her writing to help her process her experiences but she also found that seeing a good therapist was exceedingly beneficial.

"What I love about therapy is that they'll tell you what your blind spots are. Although that's uncomfortable and painful, it gives you something to work with."

https://babyology.com.au/pregnancy/stages-of-pregnancy/miscarriage/i-was-going-to-have-that-child-pink-endured-a-heart-breaking-miscarriage/

8

Never Forgotten

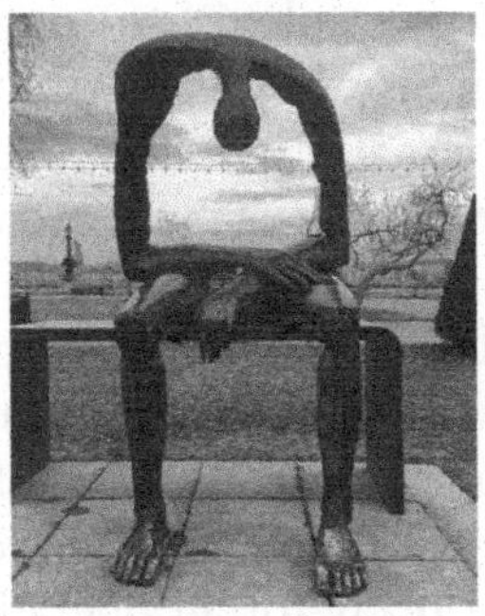

by Chelle Collins

As I write this, I find it upsetting but I'd like you to know my story. I went to my doctor in 2002 to let them know I'd done a home pregnancy test and I was in really bad pain and very sore. My so-called doctor (who had taken over from my regular doctor for the week) said I wasn't pregnant and there was no need to have a pregnancy test done. He felt my stomach; I was in absolute agony and sweating. He said he couldn't feel anything and sent me on my way.

I wasn't happy and went back one week later, to see my real doctor (who sent me for a pregnancy test and then to hospital). There, they found out I had a cyst, growing to the size of a grapefruit, on one ovary. They diagnosed me with PCOS (Polycystic Ovarian Syndrome) due to the medication (Epilim) for my epilepsy. They also said I was eight weeks pregnant. I was referred to a gynecologist and he said that when I reached twelve weeks in my pregnancy, they would operate on me to remove the cyst.

I went home but was in constant pain. I couldn't keep any food down as I was being sick constantly. Then I started to bleed, so I was back to the hospital for scans. Luckily, I didn't lose my baby and they admitted me for more tests. I came out of hospital after a few days but they kept a close eye on me.

Eventually, I woke up one morning and said to my husband, "I've lost the baby." He replied, "Don't talk daft. You don't know that." But I said, "I'm telling you I have a funny feeling I lost the baby." Call it mother's instinct. I was due to go for a scan that day so at my appointment, I told them I'd lost my baby. We went for the scan and the nurse said, "Let me go and get another nurse." Then she came back and checked the scan and said they couldn't find a heartbeat at all and they were sorry. The nurses and my husband asked, "Are you okay?" But I was numb and couldn't speak for what seemed like a good ten minutes, while staring up at the ceiling. I didn't know what to do or where to go as my head was in a whirl. I felt like my whole world had fallen apart. Then I said to the nurses, "Do it again. Do the scan again." They did, twice. Then they wanted me to go and get dressed and wait for a gynecologist to come and see me, but I asked them to do another scan in case they were wrong and they had missed the heartbeat. They did an internal scan with a light and camera on the end and then said, "Look. there is no heartbeat. We've done four scans on you now." That's when I burst into tears and felt like I was crumbling.

They put me in another room away from other pregnant women so I wouldn't upset them, even though they all saw me coming out of the room, crying. A gynecologist came in and wanted to see me. I was nine-weeks pregnant when my baby died. My gynecologist wanted me to stay in hospital that day to be ready for an operation the next but I wasn't ready; I needed to go home for the night and gather my thoughts and get my bag together. I cried all night.

The next day, I was in hospital, locking myself in a toilet, falling on the floor crying, feeling my stomach for the very last time, thinking about what could have been but somehow, wasn't to be, not wanting to come out until my husband got a nurse who could open the door.

The nurses took me in a big room and wanted me to read leaflets on my operation but I just cried and couldn't see the paperwork. My husband couldn't come into the big room with me; they made him wait in the corridors of the hospital, so I asked the nurse to read it for me as I continued to cry, with my heart aching. Then, I had to sign the paperwork with my eyes full of tears, which, somehow, I managed. They asked me to get onto a bed and took me through to the operating theatre. My gynecologist told me everything about the operation and what would happen afterwards but it was all a blur. The only thing I pleaded for was to save my ovary, as they said I might lose it because, apparently, the cyst was growing around it.

I had drips in my arm and they asked me to wear a mask and count. When I came 'round from my operation, I was shaking like mad and my head was in a whirl and at first, I didn't know where I was. The nurse told me and I calmed down, but I was still shaking from the anesthetic. I was also on morphine and felt sick and my stomach was very sore. I was put into a ward with women who'd undergone hysterectomies.

After a few days of rest, I could walk around, but it was very hard as I was bent over and could not stand up straight. The nurses were obviously telling me off and asking me to stand up and walk straight but it was hard work and my stomach felt like it was tearing apart from being so sore. I eventually managed to walk 'round but I needed help from my husband or a nurse. I had a bath but my husband had to help me on a hoist. In the bath I burst out crying and said I wanted to die.

After two weeks in hospital, they took the big white plaster cast off my stomach. It hurt; I had 38 staples in my stomach (just above the pubic bone) from my operation. Obviously, I was going to have a scar. When the gynecologist was on his rounds, he asked me questions and then said that I was allowed to go home, but not to lift anything heavy and that I needed to rest. When he left my bed to go to another patient, I asked the nurse to bring him back as I needed to talk to him. He came back and I started to tear up. I said, "Thank you for everything you have done for me; I really appreciate everything and please say, 'Thank you,' to the nurses as well." He said, "You're welcome," and that I'd go on to have more children as they had managed to save my ovary by cutting off the cyst that was around it.

When I came home, I went into a state of depression and anxiety and didn't want to go out anywhere, but my husband pulled me out of it. I went back to see my gynecologist and he was brilliant. He said the cyst had gotten to the size of a grapefruit; that's why I had been in so much pain. It had been only a few inches from the baby and it would have been squashing the baby, killing it. He said that when my baby died, the cyst had gone down to the size of a tangerine. They sent it off to the laboratory to see if it was cancerous or not. He said when they'd cut into it, they discovered it was layers of cysts inside each other with a bit of fluid in the middle but luckily, it wasn't cancerous. He also said that I could try for another baby three months after my operation, but I couldn't wait and fell pregnant two months afterwards.

I had to be under the care of a gynecologist for all of my subsequent pregnancies. I went through my second pregnancy with a cyst growing again but luckily, it went down and away after three months. As I'm epileptic, I was under the constant watch of my gynecologist, and nurses, and having scans constantly. I had all the same munchies as my first pregnancy: chips and curry and cherry tomatoes. I had morning sickness but it was worth it; I had a healthy, baby girl. I went on to have two more babies; they were both boys (I never developed any cysts with my boys). My munchies were beer and liver with both of them but being pregnant, I knew not to drink any alcohol (I drank water throughout all of my pregnancies) and I don't like liver (and it's bad for pregnancy as well). It may sound strange but because my symptoms and munchies were the same for my first two pregnancies, I know that my first baby, whom I lost, was a girl.

I'm glad my three children are all healthy; however, I will never forget my first baby. I have a scan photo of her but it has faded very badly (hopefully, I can get it restored). I am proud of the scar that I still have on my stomach; it reminds me of her every day.

Public Figures Share Their Personal Experiences To Help Others

Loni Love – *8 weeks. Unknown /Undisclosed.*

> "I just never wanted that feeling again, because I was always afraid. I had so much love for that baby. ... That's why I don't take it lightly. After that, I made sure that I would never get pregnant again, because I didn't want to have to go through that. I felt like it was a person that I was letting down...That's the reason I don't have children to this day."

https://www.refinery29.com/en-us/2017/03/146637/loni-love-miscarriage-the-real-kids-talk

9

Getting to my Rainbows

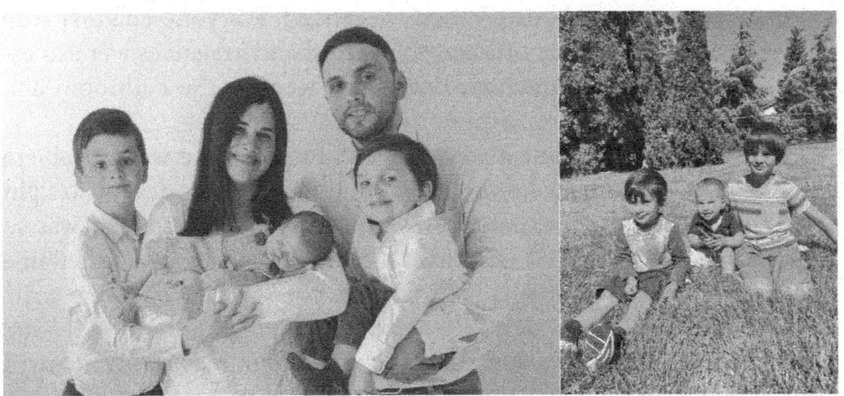

by Natasha Pandeli-Veyssiere

In 2013, my fiancé and I decided to try for a baby. Because my cycles were like clockwork, I thought it would be easy to get pregnant. The first month we tried, I fell pregnant. We were on cloud nine, but little did we know an enormous chapter in our lives was about to begin, the chapter of miscarriages, seeing countless gynecologists, fertility treatment, and almost getting cancer. This journey forced me to grow in ways I would have never imagined; it put me the through the deepest pain and brought me the greatest joy I have ever felt.

When I saw that first positive pregnancy test, I was smug. I thought, *Ha! I'm one of the lucky ones; that was so easy!* I didn't have much morning sickness; I just felt a little sleepy. I was so excited. I immediately booked an appointment with my gynecologist. We were lucky to get a dating ultrasound at six weeks. We went in so excited to see our baby. The gynecologist got the internal ultrasound ready, put it inside, and then as if it were nothing at all said, "Sorry, no baby."

I didn't understand. *How could there be no baby? I'd had a positive test. I'd felt tired.* The gynecologist explained that it was a blighted ovum.

A blighted ovum is a cruel joke; your body develops the gestational sac, and sometimes the yolk sac, but no fetus. Your body also doesn't realize that anything is wrong and you are oblivious to the fact you aren't really pregnant.

That miscarriage, my first miscarriage, was incredibly hard. Not only was I not really pregnant but my body wouldn't even miscarry; I had to go into the hospital and get a D&C. The procedure wasn't terrible because in my mind, I just wanted it over so I could try again. I knew the faster it was over, the faster I could be a mum.

Within a month, I was pregnant again. I was so excited! It surely wouldn't happen again; this time I was going to be a mum. I told all my family and started picking out names. We even decided to go on holiday to my mother-in-law's house. When we arrived, everyone couldn't stop talking about the new baby-to-be. All my husband's relatives were so excited about the first grandchild. But then I went to the bathroom and there was blood.

I was so scared. I knew it was over and I knew there was a problem with me. We rushed back home (a five-hour journey), and went straight to the ER. When we got there, I was sent to see an intern who was so nervous he was shaking. He examined me and immediately said the same thing, "There is nothing there. No baby. Are you sure you are pregnant?" I was beside myself. *How do I keep feeling pregnant, dreaming of this baby, feeling my stomach, imagining this baby, when all I am is an empty uterus?* I went home and wept.

Once it was over, we consulted a fertility specialist. I explained what had happened and they agreed it did not sound normal and that I should be checked to see if there was something wrong. This time, we waited. As we waited, I began researching. I empowered myself by understanding everything that could go wrong. I learned about female anatomy. I became obsessed. Then I came across high natural killer cells (NK cells) and I knew I had found the answer.

When you have high natural killer cells, your body thinks the embryo is an invader and kills it off like a cancer cell. The miscarriages are always early, either before a positive pregnancy test, before nine weeks, or a blighted ovum (like me). Once the placenta is formed and takes over nourishment for the baby, the NK cells can no longer do any harm.

It was time for our appointment with the fertility specialist; we were excited to finally get our answer. The gynecologist, the head of an entire gynecological hospital, tested me for a long list of things. I asked him to test me for high NK cells and he said, "No. It's not that," He said, "High NK cells don't cause miscarriages." I was so angry. I knew that was the problem and I wanted to be tested.

Instead, a few weeks later, he told me I had a very severe blood clotting disorder called protein S deficiency and needed to see a specialist immediately. He said he had never seen levels as low as mine. I thought, *Well, maybe he's right, maybe this is why I'm miscarrying.*

I was immediately seen by a hematologist. He took one look at my results and started laughing. "I'll test you again," he said, "but these are wrong. You would be dead if these results were accurate." I got tested again and he was right, my levels were totally normal. I was back to square one.

Luckily, I had already come up with a plan B. I found the only doctor in France (where I was living at that time), who specialized in NK cells. I knew that's what I had and that I would prove the other doctor wrong. I met a lovely young woman who tested my NK cell levels and sent my results to another doctor who was set to be my new gynecologist. He, too, was a lovely man. He decided to run more tests, including sperm tests on my husband. The results came back and I was right: I had high NK cells.

I was so happy. I had a reason; I could have a treatment ... I would become a mother.

We began trying again. Just a few weeks before our wedding, I was pregnant again. I was on cortisone, but not the dose I had read was necessary to reduce my number of NK cells. I was also not given intralipids (a blood infusion of fats that had been proven to lower NK cells). I begged the doctor to give me the correct treatment but he said no. (He was the doctor; he knew what was best.) I went for an early ultrasound and for the first time, my uterus wasn't empty. Inside the gestational sac was a tiny little circle with a heartbeat. I was ecstatic. It had worked; it had worked; it had worked!!

I had a beautiful, picture-perfect wedding in Paris. I couldn't have asked for it to be better.

One week later, I went for the next ultrasound. My doctor was on holiday, so I was sent to see an intern in the ER. We were so excited; we were going to see our baby again! I laid down on the table. The intern looked at me with no emotion and said, "Sorry there is no heartbeat." The baby had died the day after our first ultrasound.

The pain I felt with this miscarriage was deep. It was so cruel to have heard this beautiful little heartbeat and then be told, "Sorry, it's done." Again, my body didn't miscarry and I had to go in for a D&C.

When I went in for the procedure, the girl sitting next to me was having an abortion. I'm pro-choice but the pain I felt knowing that she could have a baby but was choosing to abort was almost unbearable. Never will I understand why they put women who are miscarrying next to those having an abortion.

My next step was getting the treatment I wanted from the best specialist for NK cells in the world. I had kept hearing about this particular researcher; I knew he was my best bet to become a mother. We decided to fly to London to meet with Doctor Shehata at the London miscarriage center.

We got an appointment quickly and I was tested. He immediately told me that my NK levels were some of the highest he had ever seen, that the dosage I had been put on during the last pregnancy wasn't enough, and that I also needed intralipids. What I had told the other gynecologist was right. Unfortunately, because I was living in Paris, I couldn't have my entire treatment in the UK. Instead, I brought all results and a letter from the doctor to my fertility specialist in Paris. Luckily, he was a very modest man and said he would follow the other doctor's treatment. He also told me he wanted to do IVF, using ICSI (intracytoplasmic sperm injection), in order to make sure everything was controlled.

A week later, I started fertility treatment. I was pumped full of drugs until I was ready. I ended up with a very high number of perfect embryos. I also ended up with hyper ovarian syndrome (my body produced so many ovules that it swelled and filled dangerously with liquid). I was told there could be serious risks if I did the transfer. I went for it anyway. Luckily, the swelling went down.

Five days later, I got a big fat positive on my pregnancy test. I was pregnant again! This time I wasn't excited, I was terrified. I couldn't go through it again. My husband and I agreed that if it didn't work, we would stop and look into adoption.

I took many pills. I injected my stomach with Lovenox. I had infusions of intralipids. The first ultrasound was just around the corner and I was more scared than I had ever been in my life. The midwife saw me and smiled, "Don't worry," she said, "It's going to go well!" I said nothing; I was trying not to cry.

In my head I kept seeing an empty sac. In reality, I saw a beautiful little embryo with a strong heartbeat. I immediately called Doctor Shehata and he said, "Fantastic! Get a nine-week ultrasound and if it's good, you are all clear." He told me that the heartbeat we had heard at six weeks with the last pregnancy wasn't strong enough, but this time, it was. I was happy but still terrified.

The nine-week ultrasound came. I was so scared I couldn't breathe. The midwife took her time; someone else had needed help. I just waited, scared out of my mind. Then she came back, put the ultrasound wand in me and turned the screen towards me. My eyes were fixed on that screen. "There you go," She said, "There is your baby." I immediately started crying my eyes out.

That was perhaps the happiest moment in my life. At that moment, I knew I was going to be a mum. I knew all my pain and suffering was for a reason. The midwife looked at me and scolded me, "Stop crying," She said. "You will scare the other patients."

After a crazy pregnancy, marked by bad morning sickness, threatened premature labor, and a uterus that wouldn't stop contracting, I gave birth to my son. The first time I held him, after my three-day delivery, I felt more joy, more pride, and more sense of accomplishment than I had ever believed was possible. He was perfect, he was mine; I had done it. The midwife that had delivered my son heard about my story and came to congratulate me. She told me stories like mine were why she loved being a midwife.

Three years went by and we were ready to try for baby number two. I still had many embryos left, so we decided to do a frozen transfer using the same treatment I had with my son. The first round didn't work and I felt defeated. *I was so fertile, how did it not work?*

Then we got pregnant naturally. I was thrilled. Immediately, I started taking my treatment and was ready to have our second child. Instead, I began to get extremely sick. My vomiting was out of control; I couldn't even keep down water. They tested my HCG and my numbers were very, very high. I was excited, am I having twins? I quickly booked an ultrasound. This time, I wasn't scared. *Surely everything was fine if my morning sickness was this bad.* Instead, when the midwife put the ultrasound wand in me she suddenly got a scared look on her face. She quickly called an OBGYN. I knew something was wrong, very wrong. The OBGYN came and told me I was having a partial molar pregnancy (when two sperm fertilize the egg at the same time). It causes the embryo to form along with a cancerous growth. This pregnancy could mean I was going to have cancer.

They immediately scheduled another D&C and removed the pregnancy. Then the testing began. I had to go for weekly blood tests to make sure my hormones were dropping. If they didn't, that would mean the cancer was spreading and I would need chemotherapy. Every week was extremely frightening. *Was I going to be free of this? Was I going to die from this?*

After a month of testing, my numbers weren't dropping fast enough. I got checked and there was something left. I was beyond petrified but I was also determined to beat it. Nobody was taking me seriously in France so I flew to a clinic in Austria that was recommended to me and I had another D&C. This time, my numbers started to go down. I had done it. I was clear of the partial molar pregnancy. I didn't have cancer; I was healthy.

I waited a month, as I was told this was necessary, and then went in for another frozen transfer. This time it worked. The pregnancy was healthy. I was thrilled. My son was going to have a brother. My second baby would be perfect.

I was so excited to see my new baby at the twenty-week ultrasound. The doctor was very nice and showed us everything. He got to the face and said, "Let's leave this and we will come back to it." When we were done, he told us that our baby was going to be born with a cleft lip and palate. We had been warned of the potential side-effects of cortisone but didn't believe it would happen to us. In any case, we didn't really have a choice – without it, I surely would have miscarried.

Our beautiful son, Elio, was born a few months later. He did have a large cleft lip and palate but he was still gorgeous. I was worried about him at birth but also completely in love with him. Luckily, we were sent to an amazing surgeon who gave him his forever smile. His story is for another time but it made me grow more than I believed a human could grow. It made me learn the true meaning of beauty. I am thankful to have been given him exactly as he is.

Life went on and we moved to Canada. COVID hit and the world stopped. We stayed indoors and waited for the curve to flatten. Nothing changed as the days went on until suddenly it did. Much to our astonishment, I got pregnant again. We weren't trying to get pregnant and so it was a huge surprise. Because of what happened to Elio, we decided I wouldn't take any medicine this time. If I miscarried, then I miscarried. So be it. We were already so blessed to have our boys and didn't need anything more in life. Well, the first ultrasound came and looking at me on the screen was a tiny circle in a gestational sac. In the middle was a very strong heartbeat. I couldn't believe my eyes! I lay there, with a mask over my mouth, all alone, (my husband wasn't allowed in the room because of COVID), thinking, *What on earth is happening? How has my body done it alone? Could it have been the fact that I was very sick two months earlier with what may have been COVID? Did the virus destroy my immune system, lowering my NK cells and preventing me from miscarrying?*

My husband was then allowed to come in to quickly look at the screen and take a picture. All he could say was, "Wow! How did this happen?" I'm now eleven weeks pregnant with severe morning sickness and a growing belly, waiting for my next ultrasound in two weeks to confirm that everything is ok. Because of COVID, I wasn't allowed my nine-week ultrasound and so I am just waiting, hoping, and vomiting.

Infertility is the biggest rollercoaster you will ever be on. Trying to survive those falls becomes your mission and getting to those rainbows in the sky becomes your dream. To anyone going through infertility or miscarriages: trust your gut; doctors don't always know everything. Never give up, and believe in happy endings.

Public Figures Share Their Personal Experiences To Help Others

Ali Wong – *Twin miscarriage. Unknown/Undisclosed.*

"It really helped me when I had a miscarriage to talk to other women and hear that they'd been through it, too. It's one thing to hear the statistics but it's another to put faces to the numbers so you stop feeling like it's your fault.

"I think that's one of the reasons women don't tell people when they've had a miscarriage -- they think it's their fault. I remember I worried what my in-laws would think, which is so crazy. I thought they'd think their son had married a terrible person."

https://www.theguardian.com/culture/2016/jun/09/comedian-ali-wong-netflix-baby-cobra-fresh-off-the-boat

My Journey to Motherhood

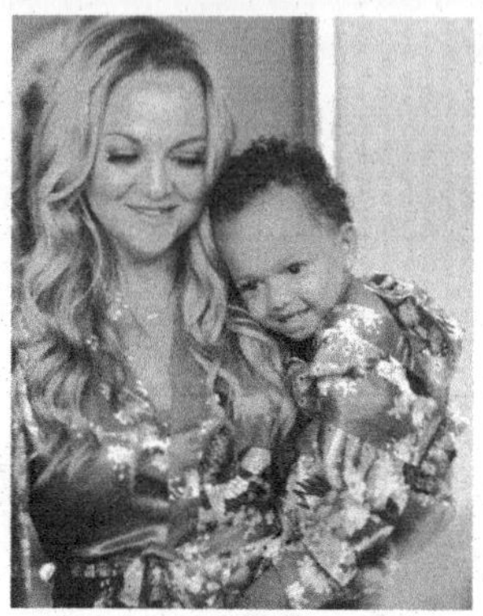

by Dana Colon

While battling a rare un-diagnosed disease, I had become pregnant. I was financially stable, a little over 32 at the time, and extremely excited. I was definitely ready; I even started to picture what he or she would look like. Then, only five short days after finding out, I woke up in the night, bleeding. I headed to the E.R. only to confirm I had lost my baby.

Just four short months later, I was diagnosed with Cushing's disease, and two weeks after that, I was in major surgery to have a tumor removed from my kidney. That was just the beginning; six surgeries later, I was on the road to recovery and healing. I wasn't allowed to try to get pregnant again for a while because I was so sick. As I healed, I still longed to be a mother.

Finally, three years later, I was allowed to start trying again, and guess what? Wow, it was a success! I got pregnant the very first month I was allowed to try since getting sick, and I was on very strong medication to heal my bones to boot! My journey to be a mother was happening, or so I thought. I was healthy and pregnant and I counted down the days to my first ultrasound, only to hear the dreadful words, "There is no heartbeat." My heart shattered into a million pieces, as did Charles'. I had to have a D&C.

After that, I became obsessed with trying to figure out what went wrong but since this was Charles' and my second loss, we were referred to a fertility specialist in Clearwater. That was the beginning of another very long journey of physical and genetic testing, which all came back good.

So, we decided to use fertility meds to expedite the trying-to-conceive process. After eight months, our reproductive doctor recommended IVF, so we began our research and planning to enter that journey to become parents through IVF.

In May 2020, I was off all fertility drugs and went to St. Pete with friends to enjoy my 37th Birthday. It was a blast! Well, after that, I waited for my cycle to start fertility meds and head to New York to start the egg retrieval process. God had other plans for us; He didn't want me to do IVF. We got pregnant naturally. My home was filled with joy. Then, the next ultrasound came. I dreaded it. This was supposed to be exciting. I was scared. I had all the symptoms, just like before, but this time, I felt uneasy and scared. Our next ultrasound was devastating, again. "There's no heartbeat." *How could this happen again? All the tests were right! My hormone levels were good!*

Fast forward to July 1st, 2020. My body was failing me again. I opted not to have a D&C and to let my baby go naturally. I did and sent him away for testing. It came back that he was a healthy, chromosomally normal baby boy. I decided to name him Baby B, for Baby Bennett. My heart and Charles' broke again in a million pieces. We were empty. My home was hollow. Baby B was perfect. *Why isn't he here!?*

But in God's timing, the best was yet to come, and it actually did come! God, in his glory, sent me my baby girl!

Two weeks after I lost my baby boy, a woman (who was a former employee of mine) sat in my salon chair and said, "I have a friend that is having a baby and we're trying to find a family to adopt her, but it has to be the right family, as the birth mother does not want the baby to go to anyone she doesn't know." Oddly enough, I had gone to middle school with the birth mother, and without any hesitation, I said, "I will take her!" I had prayed for a child for so long, I felt like this had definitely happened for a reason.

On August 13, 2020, at 7:13 a.m., my sweet baby girl came into the world. I named her Jovie Zaiya, which means, "Joyful, the Lord is gracious," and is she ever. My story wasn't pretty or easy. There was a lot of grief, depression, anxiety, and sleepless nights. I still think about my heavenly babies and wonder how they would have turned out, but I'm at peace knowing they're with the Lord, and I have no doubt that I'm meant to be Jovie Zaiya's mother.

11

My First Homebirth

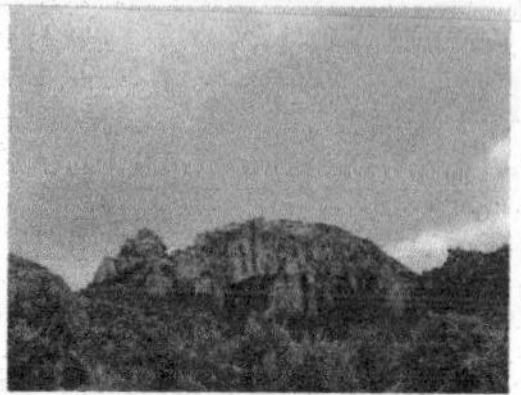

by Bee Portillo

I was three weeks pregnant when I surprised my husband, Sergio, at his office with the news about our third child. I even kept it a secret for two days, planning how I'd tell him. There is nothing like having Valentine's Day cookies made for your announcement. I even had our two little ones hand daddy the cookies.

The week Covid-19 hit, we were traveling to the Grand Canyon with our friends. Everyone and everything broke out into chaos. We headed out early in the morning on our way to Albuquerque, NM before going to Flagstaff and Sedona, AZ. We stopped at Costco in Lubbock, TX to get water, socks for my cold toes, and strawberries and blueberries for my daughter. I will always remember listening to Elevation Church online since it was a Sunday, and then listening to their worship, and the release of their new song, "The Blessing." For some reason, it captivated my heart and from then on, it set the entire mood for me throughout our trip. I could tell our baby Corban was excited about where we were. I had never been so happy, energetic, and excited to be anywhere in my life. I just knew it was him.

The spotting started when we arrived at the Grand Canyon. I was a little unsettled at first, but then I thought that it was normal to spot when pregnant. It continued throughout that day and into the next. Then spotting turned into bleeding. I knew something wasn't quite right, but I kept faith and prayed that all was okay. We got to hike The Sandia Mountains, see the Grand Canyon, along with real snow in the Coconino Forest, and the red mountains in Sedona. I was beyond the moon to be in such places as these, especially during a pandemic. We were where no one else was, so it felt that much more personal for us to see these amazing parts of the world.

We finished off seeing a very interesting abandoned village as we left Flagstaff. We were a little more than half way back to Albuquerque when I told my husband to turn back around and stop at the nearest Walgreens or CVS so I could use the restroom. I had him call one of my midwives. I was there in the restroom cleaning myself up with wipes and toilet paper, worried. So much blood was dripping. There were some clots, but none big enough. I moved everything around in the toilet bowl to see if I could see my baby or find him, in case he'd slipped out without my realizing it. He wasn't there. My midwife comforted me over the phone and said it may be normal or I may be losing him, but the only way to tell was to either go to the ER or wait until I got home to see her.

We finally made it to Albuquerque and stopped at a hotel to rest for the night. I only slept for about an hour or two and then woke up very uncomfortable with my bottom soaked in blood. I woke my husband up and told him I needed to go to the ER. I needed to see my baby on the screen and hear his heartbeat to make sure he was okay.

Thankfully, we went to a private ER with no other patients around. There we were, at one-thirty in the morning, praying and waiting for the ultrasound technician to arrive. I could tell the technician was trying to save me from heartache by not letting me see the screen and leaving the heart monitor off most of the time. As time passed, I heard no heartbeat. When he kindly let us know he was done, all I could do was cry in Sergio's arms.

They couldn't see anything. They said my body must have passed him already. But where? I never saw him. I was crushed and shocked at the same time. Sergio needed to take a breather outside on his own, to cry. It hit him hard. I felt stuck and frozen because of just how much I was in shock. I didn't want to believe it, but it was true. Our sweet baby had passed away.

On our way to my parents, I started to have really bad cramps. I was even having to breathe through them. When we finally got there, we had hugs and hot plates of food waiting for us but before we sat down to eat, I went to the restroom to check my pad to make sure I wasn't bleeding more heavily than I had been earlier. Sergio followed me in and, as I was peeing, I felt something come out of me and we both heard a different sound this time, a heavier splash. We weren't sure at first but then Sergio scooped up our baby boy out of the toilet bowl and rinsed him off. We could see his eyes, hands, what would have been his feet sticking out, and his umbilical cord still attached. Sergio got to see and feel his spine. We placed him in Gramma Helen's keepsake box, which was the perfect size. All along, it was contractions that I was having on our drive back home.

We weren't exactly sure when he had passed but we believe God took him in a way that would save us more heartache. I was ten weeks and two days along when I birthed our baby Corban, with Sergio by my side, only a few weeks away from my second trimester. Throughout our trip, he was with us. God protected him when the doctor wanted to do scrapings and we refused. God brought our baby back to us in a way we didn't think would happen. He has His reasons – and we can only trust that they are for the best, even though we may not like them.

I wasn't sure if it was normal to have a ceremony for a pregnancy loss that early. We waited almost two months to finally have a memorial for our baby since everything was shut down because of Covid. We had a granite urn made to have his keepsake box placed in and sealed.

When doing regular things around the house, being reminded that he had passed away hurt and saddened me so much; I had gotten used to thinking that I had to be careful with everything, then I would realize I didn't have him inside me anymore. I felt awkward when I'd lie on my stomach and when my husband wanted to make love because I was still torn about how I felt about my body. I had felt so much guilt and selfishness for moving forward without Corban inside me and yet, at the same time, I felt relieved that he wouldn't have to deal with this whole mess of a pandemic.

I eventually started changing my diet, receiving acupuncture, taking herbs, and even started exercising lightly. I read more of my Bible and started getting more involved in a women's ministry, which has helped me tremendously by seeing myself the way God sees me.

We decided that Corban's song would be "The Blessing." He was a blessing from God to appreciate the love for life, adventure, and family. A blessing to help Sergio and I appreciate everything God has given us: our little ones, and each other, as husband and wife.

I still miss my baby in my belly every day. His older brother looks forward to meeting him in heaven one day, his sister asks to make sure that he is safe, and his father is constantly improving himself to be a better father and husband. From the moment I found out I was pregnant, I made sure to rejoice every moment I could, with him inside me. He knew nothing except the comfort of my womb and the love from his family and friends. I am so thankful that God chose Corban for our family so that we could share his legacy of being happy and adventurous in the mountains. He has his crown first; he is safe and does not long for anything. Look at whom he is beside. He'll always be with us in our hearts.

Corban Alexander Portillo 3-21-2020

12

God's Miracles

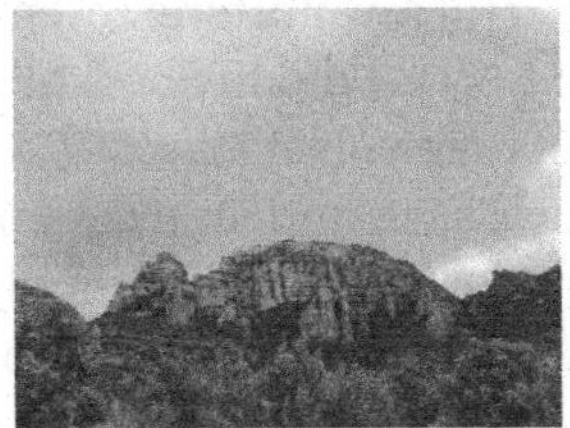

by Sergio Portillo Jr.

Corban Alexander Portillo, my little boy. Oh, son, how I wish I could've shown you the entire world! You were with us for a very short time and Jesus decided to take you home March 21, 2020. You were only about ten weeks and two days into your creation but in that short time, you managed to see the Grand Canyon, the red mountains of Sedona, and even experienced REAL snow!

Mom worked so hard to take care of you; she took her vitamins regularly, started exercising to prepare for the labor ahead, and even gave up most sugar! Big Brother was eager to show you his Jiu Jitsu accomplishments and to go exploring; sweet Sister would speak to you through mom's belly and would point and say, "Baby!" It seemed she knew you were already in there, and in this world with us, as God put you together in Mom's womb. I would helicopter over Mom, making sure she didn't do anything too strenuous or get overly stressed. We were all doing our part!

Mom became concerned; the spotting was turning into bleeding and fear started to creep in. We decided to cut the vacation a little short to let her rest; but it seems God had different plans. At nearly midnight, Mom woke me up because the bleeding had gotten worse and we rushed to the ER. I prayed over you, Corban, over Mom, your siblings, and myself. I prayed for His protection, wisdom, and understanding but most importantly I prayed for the strength to accept His will.

We wanted to hear your heart. We wanted to see your movements. We wanted to believe the faith we had been claiming would manifest itself. The doctor gave his two cents, coming from his "twenty years of experience," and used the "M" word (which I disdain) several times, speaking as if you weren't my little boy. He wanted to use invasive exams and ultimately discard you if you weren't "viable." I refused; I claimed that regardless of your state of being, your mother and I were going to place our trust in God first and go through the natural process.

The minutes turned into a couple of hours and I found myself walking in and out of the building, catching my breath, praying for strength, and forcing myself to be the rock your mother would need if the news was not what we wanted. Finally, the ultrasound guy arrived and started probing around ... I could make out nothing on the screen. He proceeded to use the internal method and I still saw nothing resembling you on the screen. Mom worried and began to cry. I did my best to calm her, while trying to hide the fact that I couldn't see you at all.

After a long ultrasound scan and an even longer wait for the report, the doctor walked in with the news: the results showed nothing in Mom's womb, not even a placental sack. The doctor proceeded to tell us that most likely, Mom had already evacuated you and the bleeding was just her body cleaning itself out. Our hearts sink. The lump in my throat felt like it was about to burst out of me and the pressure in my head from holding back tears was almost paralyzing!

I did my best to explain to big brother that you were so beautiful and perfect that God simply needed to take you to heaven and you were already with Jesus. Big brother said you were playing with Jesus, while the angels all watched and brought you presents to open. I believe he is correct; God needed another angel and you were the perfect one, Corban!

It is in your name, Corban: a blessing from God returned to God. I figured I would return you to God by raising you in church, teaching you to be a godly man, and bringing you up to be a great husband and father yourself. How badly was I mistaken; "Many are the plans in the mind of a man, but it is the purpose of the Lord that will stand." Proverbs 19:21 ESV. God's purpose for you wasn't to stay here in body but he definitely made sure you would be loved and cared for eternally in our hearts and minds.

The drive back was long; it took 13 or 14 hours, total, with stops. The entire time, Mom and I alternated recounting our experiences of you, and crying over the loss of you. Mom mentioned that she was saddened to not have known where you were or when you had gone. I claimed that day, March 21, 2020, to be your birthday. Even if you weren't with us now, you were with us for that moment.

At one point, big brother mentioned, "When Corban comes back – " I cut him off; I couldn't bear the thought. I explained that you weren't coming back; you were already with Jesus, playing and opening those gifts.

This whole time, Mom kept getting cramps and we would have to stop to make sure her bleeding was under control. Needless to say, it was a very long drive back, emotionally and physically.

When we finally got to Gramma and Grampa's house, we were greeted with warm, loving hugs, encouraging words, and plates of hot food after the long day. We had already shared the news with them early that morning. Mom went to the bathroom once more to check the bleeding and I followed shortly after. Mom asked if I could cut off the ER bracelet and I asked if she wanted to keep it or throw it out. She decided to keep it and said in a broken and teary voice, "This is the only thing I have of him."

At that exact moment, God showed His sovereignty: we heard a loud BLOOP sound as something hit the water and we both though it was more blood. I looked down and there was some bloody substance in the bowl. I asked Mom if I should get it; I don't know why, but I had a feeling this wasn't another blood clot. I scooped you up, my son. I picked you up out of that bowl and rinsed you off in the sink.

There you were, Corban!

Corban Alexander, my gift to God and protector of man, here you were! I could see your tiny little webbed toes sticking out from the sack. I could make out your beautiful little eyes, your strong back, and even the umbilical cord was still intact.

Big brother was right, Corban, you did come back! I don't know now, and I probably never will, how God hid you from that ultrasound. How did He pluck you away from Mom's womb in time to save you from a doctor who was ready to discard you? And how did He put you back? Mom's cramps during the ride back were labor cramps. She labored with you all the way from Albuquerque, NM to San Antonio, TX without even knowing it, just to deliver you here at Gramma and Grampa's!

I got to hold you, Son. I got to look upon your incredible little being; and God gave me the gift of finding peace in knowing that you were with your family.

Today is your birthday, my son, March 21, 2020. We will celebrate the short, yet adventurous life you had, every year. We will miss you every day and pray for you as you play in heaven with Jesus.

Corban, I love you so much, as does Mom, Brother, and Sister; Gramma and Grampa, Momma and Tata. You are a treasured part of our lives and we will all be better for you having come into our lives, even if only for a moment.

Corban Alexander Portillo
Conceived January 2020
Born March 21, 2020
Passed March 21, 2020

Public Figures Share Their Personal Experiences To Help Others

Mariah Carey – *Miscarriage. Unknown/Undisclosed.*

> "It kind of shook us both [her and Nick Cannon] and took us to a place that was really dark and difficult. When that happened, I wasn't able to even talk to anybody about it. That was not easy."
>
> https://www.usmagazine.com/celebrity-moms/pictures/mariah-carey-nick-cannons-coparenting-moments-over-the-years/april-2017-24/

13

The Story of Our Angel Babies

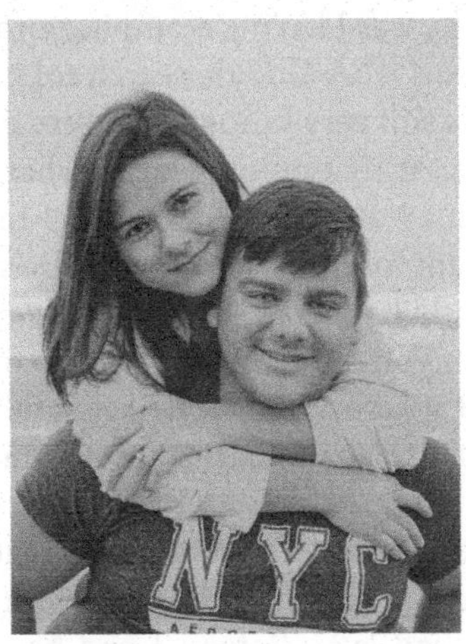

by Katie Lee

My husband and I got married in March of 2019, at ages 24 and 25. We bought a home, started our lives together, and everything seemed pretty close to perfect. We talked about our future kids at times and even discussed names for them. We both came from large families; we were both young and healthy and had no reason to think that we were going to have any trouble having kids.

Looking back, there was one thing that probably should have given me a clue that something was wrong. I had very painful periods each month, to the point where I had to leave work every time it started. But everyone seemed to pass it off as just normal period pains, and I believed them. No one ever suggested to me that there could be something seriously wrong.

We had been married for four months when we decided we were ready to grow our family. Since it was our first month trying, our expectations weren't too high, and as the time that my period was due approached, I didn't bother testing. I was feeling those familiar cramps and was sure that my period was just around the corner. The days passed and my period didn't show up. To this day, I don't know why I didn't take a pregnancy test. I think feeling all the typical PMS symptoms had me convinced I wasn't pregnant. Finally, when my period was four days late, I started having spotting and thought it was my period. I was very confused by how light it was and I was having some other unusual symptoms that confused me as well.

It was my husband who finally told me I needed to take a pregnancy test. So, I did, telling myself that I was doing it just to prove that I wasn't pregnant. But to my surprise and shock, I got a very strong positive! I was five weeks and three days along at that point. We were so excited at the thought of welcoming our own little baby into the world! But I was also very confused. Why was I having cramping and spotting? That wasn't supposed to happen, was it? A Google search told me it can be common in pregnancy, but I was still very uneasy. The very next morning, I started having heavy bleeding. At that point, I knew what was happening. I lost our baby on Sept 5, 2019 at 5 five weeks and 4 four days. We had only known we were pregnant for one day, but we were still heartbroken. I had never thought this would happen to us, especially not with our first baby.

We had not told anyone that we were pregnant, but we did tell our families afterward that we'd had a miscarriage. I felt really sad at not having had the opportunity to share that happy moment with anyone other than my husband.

We decided to keep trying to get pregnant right away. I fully believed we would get pregnant again quickly and have a healthy pregnancy. I wanted a baby more than ever. Before, I had been much more relaxed about trying, but now, I desperately wanted to be pregnant again.

My first period after the miscarriage was extremely painful. I was used to painful periods, but this was much worse than anything I had ever experienced before. I was throwing up and dry heaving for hours. My body started going numb and I was losing the ability to move. My husband was about to take me to the ER when I finally started getting some relief, so we didn't go. I did, however, make an appointment with my OBGYN, as I was convinced something was wrong.

When I finally got in to see my OBGYN, I was hoping to get some answers. I told him about the miscarriage and the painful period. He told me everything I was experiencing was normal, and that my next pregnancy was likely going to be successful. I left feeling a little disappointed but also hopeful that he was right and everything was fine.

The months passed and we didn't get pregnant quickly like I had hoped. I was disappointed time and again; but on top of that, I started dreading my periods. They continued being horrible each month and they seemed to keep getting worse (even when I thought they couldn't possibly get any worse). We even went to the ER once, hoping that we could get answers if we saw a doctor during my period but they simply did an ultrasound and told me everything was fine.

It took us six months to get pregnant again. This time, when my period didn't show up, I took a test. It was negative. I took a couple more tests over the next few days, but they were still negative; so I stopped testing and just waited for my period to show up. When it was a week late, I tested again and it was positive! I was delighted and so sure that we were finally getting our baby! This time, we simply told our families right away, since we knew we would tell them anyway if we had another loss.

However, our joy was short-lived. The very next day, I started spotting. I immediately called my OBGYN's office. They had me come in and did bloodwork and told me spotting can be normal. I was beside myself with worry, but I went home and hoped and prayed for the best. But the next morning (Feb 25th), I woke up with heavy bleeding. I had more bloodwork done that confirmed my levels were dropping and I was miscarrying again. I was five weeks and four days again according to my last cycle, but I believe that I probably was not that far along since I had gotten such a late positive.

Again, my O-GYN told me that this was probably just a fluke and that statistically, my next pregnancy was likely to be successful. He told me that because I'm young, and the miscarriages were happening so early, he wasn't worried about there being any heath issue causing them. He did say my progesterone was low but he didn't believe that was causing the miscarriages. By this time, I was getting really tired of being told the same thing over and over again. There were too many similarities between my miscarriages for me to believe that they were both just random bad luck. I asked him if I could get testing done to see if something specific was the problem. He said he would check my thyroid levels, but he saw no need to do more testing unless I had a third loss. I struggled with that. I hated the idea of having to go through another miscarriage before I could get answers.

In many ways, that second miscarriage was much harder than the first. I no longer believed it to be just a fluke and I kept wondering if we were ever going to get our baby. I also felt alone. I had friends that'd had a miscarriage, but most of them went on to have healthy pregnancies afterwards. I started connecting online with some other women who'd had experiences similar to mine. It helped me to see that I was not the only one going through this; in fact, I met many people who had suffered much more and somehow kept going.

My husband and I decided to take the following month off from trying while we waited for my thyroid test to come back. When my test came back normal, and I experienced yet another excruciating period, I knew it was time for a change. I couldn't keep going like this. I decided it was time to switch doctors. I found an OBGYN that worked with a lot of high-risk pregnancies and scheduled an appointment.

My first appointment was just a phone conversation since, by then, we were in the middle of quarantine with Covid-19. I was actually relieved to not have to face her in person, as I had tears running down my face during almost the entire phone call. Someone was finally listening and willing to help me find answers. When I told her my symptoms, she immediately suggested that I might have endometriosis. I barely knew what endo was at that point but at least I had some possible answers. My doctor told me the only way to diagnose it was through surgery and during that time, due to Covid, she couldn't do any surgeries that weren't an emergency so that had to be put on hold. She did have me come in and do a lot of bloodwork to test for other possible reasons for the miscarriages.

A couple weeks after switching doctors, I found myself with another positive pregnancy test. My new doctor started me on progesterone and baby aspirin immediately and I was very hopeful that this was going to be what I needed to make a pregnancy work. I also tested positive earlier than I ever had before, at three weeks and five days. This pregnancy felt different from the others and that gave me a lot of hope, at first.

However, in the days that followed, I started having a lot of cramps. And then I started getting this really, really sick feeling in my stomach. Most people I talked to tried to tell me it was just normal pregnancy sickness, but I knew that what I was feeling was not typical. I just knew that something was very wrong. I still tried to hold on to hope and told myself that maybe everything was going to be fine. We kept praying. But a week after finding out I was pregnant, I started spotting. Again, I was told spotting can be normal, but at that point, I just felt like I knew what was happening. A few days later, on May 6th (which also happened to be my due date for my first pregnancy), I miscarried at five weeks and one day. I remember feeling so low. This day was supposed to have been a happy day as we welcomed our first baby into our home, but instead, we were losing our third.

The days and weeks that followed were a very painful season in my life. Everywhere I looked there seemed to be pregnant women or women with babies. Pregnancy announcements were constantly popping up on social media. More than ever, I found myself connecting with people who had similar experiences. That was one of the biggest things that helped me through this third time, just being able to talk to people that understood, people who didn't say things like, "At least you can get pregnant," or, "At least it happened early;" or the seemingly innocent, but painful question, "When are you having kids?"

Shortly before the miscarriage, we had gotten all the results back from my bloodwork and everything looked great. There was nothing that should have caused any problems with staying pregnant. I was getting desperate for answers.

By this time, hospitals were starting to open up again after quarantine, so I asked my doctor if we could go ahead with the surgery to check for endometriosis. We scheduled a laparoscopy for about two weeks out. In the days leading up to it, I often wondered if I was doing the right thing. I had no proof that I had endo. I had some symptoms of it, but not all the typical symptoms. I worried that I was going to have surgery for nothing. But I had to know, and I couldn't continue having these horrible periods each month. So, on May 21st, I had the laparoscopy done. I had stage three endo, most of which was removed during surgery. It had destroyed my right tube, so that had to be removed, too. I was pretty shocked to wake up from anesthesia and learn that I had lost a tube. However, when my doctor told me that my tube was filled with toxic fluids that could kill a fertilized egg, and I saw pictures of how swollen and misshapen it was, I knew I was better off without it.

The first day or two after surgery was painful, but after that, I had a smooth recovery. It felt surreal to me to actually have received a diagnosis, as I was so used to being told there's nothing wrong with me, and being left with no answers. While on one hand I was relieved at having an answer, I was also not sure if I could ever trust my body again. I didn't feel ready or confident to try to get pregnant again. I felt like it would only result in more disappointment and heartbreak, and more things going wrong. *What if the endo kept spreading and I kept having miscarriages? What if I had an ectopic pregnancy and lost my last tube?* It took some time, and some deep conversations with my husband, before I felt like I wanted to try again. Thankfully, by the time we were given the green light by my doctor, I was feeling better about it.

We started trying again and, two months later, I was pregnant once more. I was scared and excited all at the same time. I struggled with anxiety, and felt like I was just waiting for something to go wrong. I was waiting for a phone call from my doctor to say my levels weren't increasing, waiting to start bleeding. And when I started spotting, I lost all hope and was sure I knew what was coming. But, for the first time in my history of pregnancies, the spotting stopped and everything seemed to continue going smoothly. My HCG levels were rising appropriately, and at six weeks, we saw a good heartbeat on ultrasound. I was so nervous before my ultrasound and so happy and excited afterwards. I had never gotten to see any of my babies on ultrasound before, so I started to relax just a little and believe that maybe I would meet this baby. I still had to fight doubts and anxiety every day, but I finally stopped expecting bad news at every turn. I was determined to enjoy my pregnancy, no matter how long or short it was, and I found that some little things, like talking to the baby, or journaling helped me stay positive, and eased the anxiety a little.

As the days and weeks passed, everything seemed to be going really well. And then around ten weeks, I had a little bit of spotting again, and I started to feel increasingly anxious. No matter how hard I tried to convince myself that everything was fine, I couldn't shake the feeling that my baby wasn't alive anymore. I finally scheduled a private ultrasound at a pregnancy center, hoping I would find my baby still healthy and growing and be able to relax again.

The morning of my ultrasound, I was a ball of nerves. I was counting down the hours and minutes to when I'd know if my baby was okay or not. I took a "bump photo" (even though I didn't have much of a bump), before I left home, wondering if it would be my last picture with this baby. The drive to the pregnancy center seemed unendingly long but I finally got there. It was time for the ultrasound. I got to see my baby on the screen again. But it was so, so still. There was no little, flickering heartbeat like there had been before. The sweet lady doing the ultrasound searched for a heartbeat for a long time, but I knew that my baby was in heaven with its siblings. When she turned the sound on to listen for a heartbeat, there was only a quiet, whirring sound. It seemed like the most haunting sound I had heard in my life. The baby was only measuring eight weeks when it should have been eleven.

I somehow got through the rest of the day. I called my husband and told him. I hated having to deliver such painful news to him. I knew that he fully believed everything was going to be fine; and he had tried to assure me of that many times. I heard his cheerful voice when he answered the phone and my heart sank. I desperately wished I could tell him that he had been right and our baby was fine. Instead, I knew I was about to break his heart by telling him our baby had died.

After calling my husband, I contacted my doctor. We decided to go with a D&C and do fetal genetic testing. I had another ultrasound with my doctor just for confirmation. A week later, on October 1, 2020, I had the D&C. I would have been twelve weeks along on that day. It also happened to be my 27th birthday. Needless to say, it was not my happiest. I went through the day just feeling numb and not allowing myself to feel all the emotions that were just underneath the surface.

The physical part of recovery was fairly easy and painless. Emotionally, it wasn't so easy. I was shocked a couple days after the D&C when I realized my milk had come in. I had no idea that would happen and I was devastated that my baby wasn't here to be fed.

Two weeks later, we got the results of the fetal tests. Our baby was a perfect, healthy little girl. No abnormalities were found, and there was no explanation as to why we lost her.

We hadn't known her gender while we were pregnant, but my husband and I both felt like she was a girl for the entire pregnancy. I was relieved to find out we were right, as it helped me to feel the connection I had with her was real.

It has been three weeks since the D&C. Some days, the pain feels overwhelming and I don't know how to keep going. I still miss my little girl so much, and my three other babies too, but I believe that I will see them again, and I look forward to that day.

I've realized that I really need to heal emotionally before we try to get pregnant again. Right now, just the thought of being pregnant fills me with anxiety, and I know that I won't be ready to try again anytime soon. I've joined a pregnancy loss support group and I'm just focusing on healing before we make a plan to move forward. I don't know what the future holds at this point, but all I can do is keep taking one day, one moment at a time, believing that God still has a plan for us far greater than we can see right now.

14

Zoe Grace

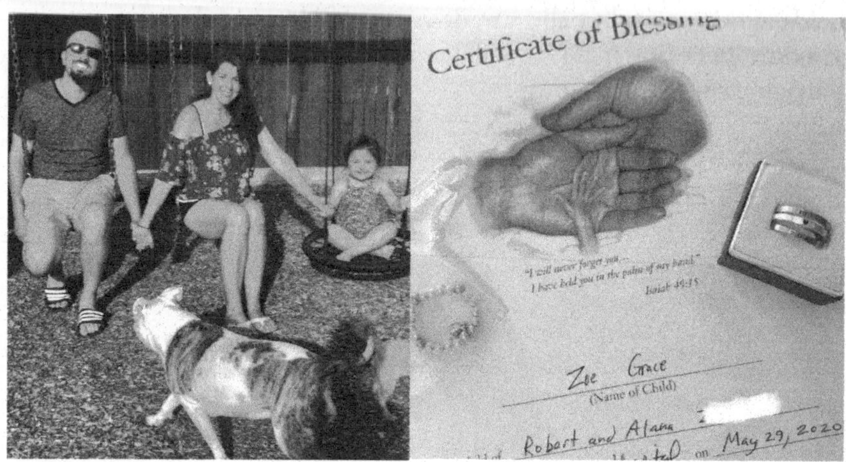

Alana Zoufal

I was 36 when I had my first miscarriage. It was January, 2016. I knew I was pregnant before any test result could tell me I was. I knew by how my body looked and felt. I took a pregnancy test and it came up negative. I called the doctor's office and was told it was early so I should wait one week and then take another. The day I took my second pregnancy test, also negative, I began bleeding. When I called the doctor's office, they didn't believe me. They told me it was just my period and that it was late. I knew they were wrong.

A little over a week later, I called to tell them I was still bleeding and I knew I had been pregnant and it was a miscarriage. They told me to come in and take a pregnancy test. Of course, that pregnancy test came up negative. I felt so alone and so stupid. I started to question myself. *Maybe I was crazy. Maybe I wasn't pregnant. The tests were all negative so I must be crazy. What if this was my only chance to be a mom?* I was sad I had lost my baby, yet I questioned the validity of what I knew was true. After bleeding for seven weeks, and a few calls to the doctor's office, I asked if I needed a D&C. They said, "No."

Eventually, half way into March, the bleeding stopped, but the following months were anything but normal. From March to July, I called several times indicating something was wrong. I bled every time we had sex and the blood had an unusual smell. I was told, "Blood smells so that's not a problem." I knew it was off, though. I told them multiple times I felt like I had an infection. I was prescribed a cream to use internally. I was told that wearing stretch pants to work was causing my infections. After months of being told I was fine and being given an explanation for everything, I continued to doubt myself. I knew something wasn't right but the nurses were not listening.

June came and I asked to see the doctor. I was told that if I was still having problems come July to let them know. July rolled around, I called and, finally, they gave me an appointment. In August, I went in to see the doctor. It took less than 30 seconds from the time the doctor started my internal exam for him to push back his chair with concern and say, "As your doctor, I am telling you, you need to have a D&C." In that moment, I remember feeling that the way he said it to me was like he had told me to get a D&C before and I had refused, which wasn't true. I reminded him that I had asked about a D&C in March and was told I didn't need one. He repeated, "You need to have a D&C." He asked if I was actively trying to get pregnant because there was no way for me to get pregnant until they completed the D&C. Due to starting a new job and needing new insurance to begin, I didn't have my D&C until October, 10 ten months after my miscarriage. Two weeks after my D&C, we conceived our daughter, who was born in July, 2017.

I was forty years old when I had my second miscarriage. After our daughter was born, we decided not to have any more children because she was Coombs positive. She had Hemolytic Disease of the Newborn due to ABO incompatibility. She was extremely sick and had many health problems after birth. We agonized over whether we should have another baby or not. Our pediatrician told us that only ten percent of babies with HDN have a severe reaction and that our daughter was on the top end of that ten percent. He told us our next baby would have it worse and that the long-term effects we were concerned about with our daughter were more likely to occur. I grieved over our decision not to have another baby. I cried. I cringed every time someone asked us if we were having another baby. Having to explain our decision each time made my heart ache with grief over the decision we had made. It was what was best for our family but that didn't make it hurt any less.

In December of 2018, I started having a lot of problems. I swore I was pregnant but I had an IUD so how could I be? Multiple pregnancy tests over three weeks kept coming up negative. I knew my body; something wasn't right. The doctor removed my IUD and put me on a gluten-free, dairy-free diet but none of that took away the recurring, extreme bloating I was experiencing or the problems with my period and bleeding. In June 2019, I cried because, once again, I had a doctor (not the same as my first miscarriage) who wasn't hearing me. I begged for hormone testing.

Everything came back ok except for one, which they attributed to taking my blood during the wrong day within my cycle. They also indicated that if we wanted to have another baby, we would need a fertility specialist because I had a very low egg reserve for my age. Since we weren't planning on having any more children, this was of no concern.

Nine months later, in January 2020, I had found a new OBGYN because we had moved. I called for an appointment for an IUD. They couldn't get me in until March. Around the same time, I started having some hot flashes. Odd things started to happen and I swore I was going through early menopause. I kept telling my friends and comparing notes. In March 2020, the Covid pandemic happened. My doctor appointment was canceled since it was a non-essential appointment.

My husband and I are special education teachers. When the pandemic hit, our schools closed, our daughter's daycare closed, and the three of us were thrown into e-learning together at home. This meant our days were filled with teaching students by video and talking with parents. It meant that nights, after our daughter was in bed, were spent creating lessons, tutorials, and interactive materials for our students and families. I was exhausted; I didn't feel well, but I thought it was because I was working so much. I had an excuse for every symptom.

It wasn't until the end of April, 2020, when my student teacher mentioned she had her period, that my mind woke up. I was so busy with teaching and e-learning and taking care of our daughter while working that I realized I hadn't had a period since February. I took a pregnancy test and it was positive. We were shocked. We took three more, all positive. I was happy and terrified all at the same time due to our daughter's experience with HDN. I immediately called my new doctor and told them I was ten to twelve weeks pregnant. They made an appointment for more tests a week later.

I was scared, I was happy; I was still in shock. Unfortunately, due to the pandemic, I had to go to the appointment alone. I went in for my ultrasound and asked if I could FaceTime my husband on the phone so he could be there virtually. The tech was apprehensive but allowed it, indicating that she would only play the heartbeat for a few seconds for us. I got the first glimpse of our baby and heard the heartbeat. I felt so bad my husband had to see it through a phone.

The pandemic really changed everything. They confirmed that I was eleven weeks pregnant but that the baby was three weeks behind in growth. Our daughter had also been three weeks behind in growth so we were not concerned. My biggest concern was the ABO incompatibility. I had read studies that you can miscarry at twenty weeks due to the ABO incompatibility. I was cautiously optimistic. We didn't tell our daughter;

we were waiting for that twenty-week appointment with our maternal-fetal medicine doctor.

The next couple of weeks were exciting, filled with so many emotions. My husband quickly went on to talking about names, talking about our future with two babies, and moving furniture around in the house. We were so excited! We continued to pray that we would have a safe and healthy pregnancy and delivery for our baby. We saw our pregnancy and our baby as a gift from God.

I was sitting in a chair folding laundry; I bent forward in just the right position to feel the first flutter of our baby. It was the most amazing feeling; I'll never forget it. I got into the position again. Again, I felt the little flutter. We had a strong baby. I couldn't stop smiling. Over the next week, I felt the baby one more time. All our genetic testing was done and came back great! We were feeling good. Then I started spotting.

I'd had spotting throughout my pregnancy with our daughter. I called the medical office; they weren't concerned. The next few days were great and then I had some back pain and more spotting so I went to bed and put my feet up. We'd had family over that day for my dad's birthday and it was Labor Day, so I thought I had just done too much. I'd had placenta previa with our daughter so I had an answer and excuse for all of it. That Tuesday, we heard from the doctor. We were having a girl. My husband and I were so excited! Two girls! It was perfect. We had all the clothes already! I pictured our daughters growing up together and hoped they would grow up as best friends.

The following night, I started to have really bad back pain and more bleeding. Thursday morning, I called the doctor's office and they had me come in for an ultrasound that afternoon. Again, I had to go alone. My husband wasn't allowed to come due to the pandemic and the hospital's rules. I sat in the waiting room looking at maternity clothes online and planning out the next few months of pregnancy. When I went in for my ultrasound, I told the tech I was sure it was just placenta previa or something. I had an external ultrasound and then an internal.

Where I previously saw my baby's heartbeat, I now saw a flatline on the screen. We had lost our baby girl. The tech apologized and told me she no longer had a heartbeat. I was alone, without my husband, and I was heartbroken. My husband was waiting in the car with our daughter, who was sleeping. I called him and just started crying. I couldn't even talk. I had to tell him over the phone while I waited for the doctor to come in. Once the doctor came in, I told my husband I would call him back. It was a doctor I hadn't seen before. She very quickly said, "I'm sorry. I heard," and then continued talking. I stopped her and asked if she could wait for me to call my husband so he could hear. Twice I asked and twice I was told, "No." She said, "I'm just going to give you a bunch of information.

You can tell him later." She went on to tell me that I probably lost the baby because I was forty and my eggs weren't viable. I said, "It's my fault we lost her?" She said, "No. Your eggs aren't viable because of your age." At that point, I stopped listening. I just kept crying. She told me at this point that since I hadn't miscarried, I'd need a D&C the following day. I was sent home with no information of what to expect other than a call for scheduling. I was devastated. As I left the hospital, I was met with the most compassionate nurses and staff. A nurse even walked me out so I wouldn't have to take that walk to my husband alone.

That night, the cramping and pain began. I told my husband I thought I was going to start miscarrying. The bleeding was getting worse. I went to the restroom and passed an extremely large mass. I was terrified that my baby was in it; I was afraid to flush her down the toilet. We used a Solo cup to scoop it out, run water on it, and look for the baby. I didn't know what to do. I was so scared. I called the doctor's office and explained what had happened. I explained that I was bleeding a lot and wasn't sure what to expect. A nurse said I should speak with the doctor. The doctor I saw earlier in the day got on the phone and said, "I'm getting ready to leave. What do you need?" She was short with me, rude, and barely answered my questions. I was told to flush the mass down the toilet and that if I bled through more than three pads an hour, I needed to go to the E.R. I asked if I should call them or just go in. I was told to just go in.

The contractions became harder. I didn't realize, and no one had told me, you literally go into labor. The back contractions. The stomach pain. I was bleeding and passing a lot of clots. Late that night, we had to go to the E.R. because my bleeding was so bad. Upon entering the E.R., we were told that my husband couldn't come with me due to Covid. I was scared, sad, and in pain, and I had to do it alone. The E.R. nurse practitioner and nurse were so sweet. They kept telling me I wasn't alone and they understood how hard it had to be to go through this without my husband. My husband sat in the parking lot in his truck and waited until four A.M.

The hospital finally said they were admitting me because I needed D&C on Friday and couldn't wait until Saturday, as scheduled. They were admitting me because I was losing a lot of blood. I was getting light-headed and kept passing clots. They came and gave me a rapid Covid test before they could admit me. I asked if my husband could come be with me. The nurse practitioner made a couple of calls thinking someone would allow it, but they said, "No." At that point, they talked me into starting pain meds. I was afraid to take anything and be out of it without my husband there, so they started me on a very low dose of morphine, which didn't do much.

I was moved up to a floor and admitted, still contracting, still sad, still alone and scared. The nurse and CNA on the floor were compassionate and kind. A few hours later, there was a nursing shift change at seven A.M. That's when things became lonelier. The day-nurse and CNA rarely came into my room. The nurse wouldn't give me my pain meds because she said I would have my D&C soon. I was listed as a fall risk because I was getting light-headed and they were supposed to check for the amount of blood I was losing. When I would call for someone, I felt like I was an inconvenience. The two times my nurse came into my room, she had me climb behind my own bed to unplug my IV; she wouldn't help me. She also left once I was in the bathroom. I had no one. I was so alone. I lay in that room with the TV off, praying and just trying to breath through the pain.

I video FaceTtimed with my husband – who was at home with my parents, taking care of our daughter. It wasn't the same. I needed him with me and he couldn't be. I kept telling myself I was strong and could do it on my own. Finally, late that afternoon, they told me I'd be going for my D&C and my husband could be with me. I went to pre-op and my husband was finally there! That lasted all of about twenty-five minutes. When it was time for me to go in for the D&C, we were told he should go back home because he couldn't be with me in recovery or back in my hospital room. I was going to be alone again.

When I woke up, I was being wheeled to recovery. I grabbed my nurse's hand, crying, asking if they had found my baby. I couldn't stop crying and fearing that I had flushed my baby down the toilet. The minister came in and immediately prayed with me. I could hear a nurse talking; telling me it was okay to feel sad and cry. The minister then asked if I had held my baby yet. I said, "No. I can't because she's too small." She told me I could and I heard her ask the nurse for my baby. I was still coming out of anesthesia and my vision was still fuzzy. I put my hands out expecting to hold a tiny, fourteen-week-old baby in my one hand, but I was handed a sealed basin, wrapped in a towel. I was so confused and disappointed; I just cried, holding this plastic tub. I listened to the prayer from the minister for our Zoe Grace. It wasn't Zoe I was holding, it was a plastic tub. As soon as the minister left, I handed the tub to the nurse and just wept. The nurses kept telling me they were sorry my husband wasn't with me, but they were there for me.

I was moved up to my room again. As they wheeled me in, I saw the day nurse (the one that wouldn't come near me or help me). She pulled a chair next to the bed, which I thought was odd considering she had avoided my room and me all day. This was the same woman who made me climb behind my bed, light-headed, contracting, miscarrying, to unplug my own IV. Yet she was sitting in a chair next to me. I quickly realized she was probably supposed to be monitoring me. When the other people left the room, she asked me why I had a D&C. I told her I miscarried. I know she knew that. It was in my records all day and the night nurse had told her during her report. She responded by asking if I had any other children.

I said, "Yes. One." She said, "Oh okay. You're okay then." Then she got up and walked out of my room. That was it. That was the extent of the conversation. I just wanted to go home and be with my husband.

Several hours later, she walked in and said I was going home. I told her I thought I was supposed to eat and drink before I left. She responded, "Did you do that?" I said, "No, because no one brought it to me even though I heard someone order it." She wasn't happy. For whatever reason, she wanted me out of there. I hadn't been a problem. I didn't complain. I only called when I needed to use the restroom. I was quiet and tried to just pray and zone out the entire time I was there. I didn't even turn on the TV. I just prayed and breathed through the experience. I didn't understand why this nurse wouldn't come near me. She wouldn't even check how much blood I had lost. She wouldn't go near the restroom. Now she was acting like it was me that was holding up my departure. Finally, I got home, in my own bed, in the arms of my husband, where I had needed to be the entire time.

In the days following my miscarriage, I was increasingly sad, angry, and hurt. During the time I was in the hospital, alone, without my husband because of Covid, elements of our society were encouraging crowds of people to be out in the streets, together, protesting – during Covid. My husband couldn't be with me; our baby was gone, and I had to be alone. But thousands of strangers could stand, side by side in protest. They could be violent, they could destroy communities, they could come together at public funerals, but my husband couldn't be with me to say goodbye to our daughter. They couldn't give my husband a rapid Covid test so he could be with me, but they were offering free Covid tests to protesters. Men could be with their wives who were in labor and delivering their live babies, but my husband couldn't be with me as we lost our daughter.

I saw our society from an entirely different viewpoint. I was let down and felt so alone in a time I needed love and support. I was grieving the loss of our daughter and the destruction of our society. Every time I saw, "Black Lives Matter," I heard, *Your daughter's life doesn't matter.* I felt like the hospital and society didn't think our daughter's life mattered or our experience mattered because I was left to do it alone. The same rules don't apply. So, I kept saying, "All lives matter." That included my daughter, who was only 14 fourteen weeks old. My life and the experience I went through mattered. Yet, I kept hearing society tell me, *She doesn't matter because she is white and because she was at fourteen weeks gestation.* My heart was filled with so much grief. I felt let down by our society.

I started to question why people see the death of a baby as just a miscarriage. Why don't we say, "My baby died. My baby passed away."? Do we use the word miscarriage to make it somehow not what it is? Our baby died. Why is it something for which we are discouraged to grieve? Why do people act like it was a cut on the arm, something a couple should just keep moving through? Why don't we ask how the dad is feeling and remember he experienced a loss, too? Our daughter died. I've had other friends go through miscarriages at many different stages. Some of them grieve openly, some grieve privately, and some never talk about it and seem to just move on.

To help myself think through it, I talked to my husband about why people don't talk about miscarriage or the loss of their baby openly. Is it fear of judgement? Fear that others will judge your grief based on how far along you were? Fear that people will judge how you are grieving? Fear that others will think you're looking for attention? For me, it's all of those things. But I also know that I am not ashamed of the hope we had for our daughter whom we loved and lost. I have a lot of feelings but shame is not one of them. We only had Zoe Grace for fourteen weeks but we will hold her in our hearts forever.

Public Figures Share Their Personal Experiences To Help Others

Nicole Kidman – *Ectopic pregnancy and a miscarriage around 3 months. Unknown/Undisclosed.*

"From the minute Tom and I were married, I wanted to have babies. And we lost a baby early on, so that was really very traumatic. And that 's when it came that we would adopt Bella."

https://www.closerweekly.com/posts/nicole-kidman-tom-cruise-miscarriages-161019/

"I know the yearning. That yearning. It's a huge, aching yearning. And the loss! The loss of a miscarriage is not talked about enough. That's massive grief to certain women.

"There's an enormous amount of pain and an enormous amount of joy on the other side of it. The flip side of going through so much yearning and pain to get there is the feeling of 'Ahhhh!' when you have the child."

"Whether you're an adoptive mother, whether you're a foster mother, whether you're a biological mother – it's the emotion of attaching to a child and helping to guide them and rear them [that is important].

"[Getting pregnant] was a miracle because I'd not thought I'd be able to have [a baby] in my lifetime. I'd had a lot of complications, and I don't mind speaking about it because I think it takes the onus off it [for other women].

"They told me I was probably not going to be able to have a child, a birth child. It was, 'OK, that's it.' And then, out of blue ... And that was Sunday. Sunday Rose appeared. So that's a very, very powerful thing to happen."

https://www.tatler.com/article/nicole-kidman-tatler-interview

Public Figures Share Their Personal Experiences To Help Others

Carrie Underwood & Mike Fisher – *Three Miscarriages (around 2 to 3 months). Unknown/Undisclosed.*

Mike: "Well, you definitely learn a lot as a parent. Five years into our marriage, we had Isaiah. and We had this awesome gift and then we wanted him to have a little brother or sister and we start[ed] planning (as we all do in our mind[s])."

Carrie: "I'm a planner. I like to know what's happening all the time."

Mike: And "We get pregnant again, fairly easily, and, um, you know, months in, we lose, lose the baby. And it's obviously a fear?" He makes it a question as he looks over to his wife. "It was a fear for you."

Carrie: "It sounds wrong when you say it, but it's one of those 'bad things that happens to other people,' you know what I mean? It's like so many things in the world: it's not something that you ever envision yourself having to deal with."

Mike: "You know, it was time, and We try again and we get pregnant right away again and uh, months into it, same thing. And uh You pray and you pray and you pray… And um Sometimes, I think I'm guilty of expecting God to be a genie in a bottle and its [He's] not that, and your trying [thinking] *Ok, why is this happening?* And you don't know why and sometimes you will never figure out why."

Carrie: "Mike came to me one day and said, um, 'We're going to have another baby and it's going to be a boy and his name's going to be Jacob.' And I was like, 'Ok, and you know this because?'"

Mike: "I was frustrated; we'd had two miscarriages. *What's the future look like? We don't know. Are we going to adopt? Are we going to* … going through things in your mind. And I was just kind of wrestling, and probably the most honest I'd been with God ever in my life and I heard, not audibly, but I just heard … I just sensed that God told me that we were going to have a son and his name's Jacob. Not much longer, we were pregnant and we lose another baby and I remember you [Carrie] coming to me."

Carrie: "I was just like, *Where is he? Where is he?*"

Mike: "And I was like, *Oh well, I guess,* I guess, you know *God didn't,* you know … *Was I hearing things right?* So we get pregnant again and, I think it was a Friday night, she [Carrie] was like, 'I lost the baby,' and I was like, I was like, 'There's no way, again?' I was like, 'Well, you don't know.' And you [Carrie] were like, 'Yeah, I know.' Called your doctor, and the doctor was, 'Yeah, it's not good.'"

Carrie: "He," Carrie gestures to her husband, "was gone the next day and uh, I'd just kind of had enough. I just remember kind of just not wanting to be by myself, so I uh went up to Isaiah's room and crawled into bed with him. And I don't know how that kid didn't wake up because I was bawling.

"I feel like I've been a Christian my whole life. I always wanted to be a good daughter and you know, having a child, it's like even if you know what's wrong with your child, you want them to talk to you about it; you want to make that connection. And I just had an honest conversation with God and I told him now I felt: I was hurt, I was a little angry (of course you feel guilty for being mad at your creator), and I told him I needed something, I needed; we needed to have a baby or not ever because like I couldn't keep going down that road anymore.

"Monday, I text my doctor, 'Can I just come in so we can just see and um I can close the door and move on?' And a couple hours later, the nurse called me, and I felt like she was surprised, like she wasn't even expecting to tell me what she was going to tell me. And she told me my, my numbers, my levels, were like weren't just where not just where they were supposed to be but like way past, through the roof, no doubt about it, all looks good! And we went in later on that day and had an ultrasound. And it's like its all ok; everything is ok. So we were like, 'Jacob this is Jacob.'"

Mike: "Yup. For the longest time, I didn't really know why 'Jacob' either."

Carrie: "It wasn't ever a name that we had talked about."

Mike: "No, we'd never. And the story of Jacob: he wrestled with God through the night and he wouldn't let him go until he got his blessing. We weren't demanding that He gave us His blessing; we were just being honest with him. Jeremiah 29:13 says, 'You will seek me and find me when you seek me with all your heart.' It's so true. So many times, you're on the mountain tops and things are great and sometimes those are the hardest times because you don't feel like you need God but then, you go through the valleys and you actually really seek Him and His will and that's when you learn and grow and He changes you. He changes our marriage for the better. We're able to kind of work though our faith together like we had never done before, for sure."

Web Series: Mike and Carrie: God & Country, https://www.youtube.com/watch?v=JSc4StfnPAo

15

Three Butterflies

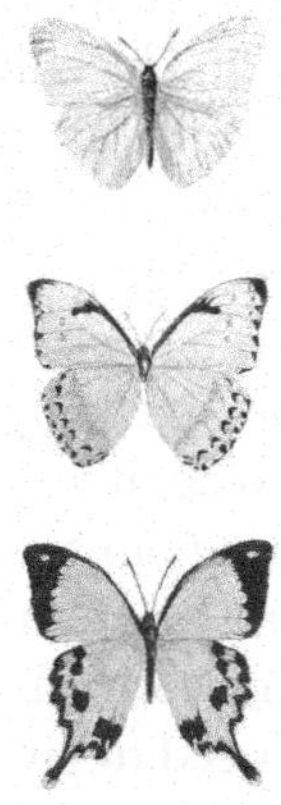

by Y. Jordan

I always pictured myself having a family one day. When I married my husband, we decided we would start trying for a baby after being married for a year. A little over a year passed and, unexpectedly, I found out I was pregnant. I was in shock; I was scared, happy, excited, and my whole life changed in an instant. I felt so lucky; I was going to be a mom. We were so happy.

As the weeks went on, I had a stressful early pregnancy (though all of my blood work was great). When I was seven weeks pregnant, I traveled down to Florida to visit my sister and my nieces and nephew. We stayed by the beach for a few days. I woke up one morning cramping and bleeding. I showed my sister the blood from when I wiped and her face scared me. She wanted to take me to get looked at but with my flight a few hours away, I just wanted to get home. I proceeded to fly home to Chicago. I cried the whole flight. I was sure that I was having a miscarriage. As I arrived home, the bleeding stopped and I visited the doctor, where he assured me my cervix was closed and it was probably just an early pregnancy bleed. I found myself wondering, *How many women was I ever next to in a bathroom stall going through that?* It was a scary experience but I remained hopeful.

We had a normal ultrasound at nine weeks. When I saw my baby and this tiny heart beating inside of me, it was the best feeling I can ever remember. We just couldn't wait any longer; we were so excited to share the news with our family and friends, so we did.

Fast-forward two weeks; it was August in Chicago and we went up to Lake Geneva for a weekend getaway, which is about an hour and a half from the city. I had some cramping that day but I figured it was just growing pains. A few hours later, I started bleeding and the pain started. I was a little over 11 weeks. I called the doctor's answering service and they told me to head to the closest emergency room. When I explained my symptoms to the doctor, I will never forget her saying to me, "You still have time to drive back to the city if you leave now." So, we headed back to my hospital where I was seen immediately. By this time, there was so much blood I didn't even know what to do. It was, to this day, the most pain I've ever experienced. I ended up losing most of the tissues and my baby there. The whole experience is still kind of a blur. I just remember being curled up in the hospital bed and crying so hard I couldn't breathe. The doctor that took care of me said, "You need to give yourself time to grieve." And she hugged me. I thought to myself, *Grieve?* It still hadn't hit me.

After hours of being there, we came home and somehow fell asleep for a few hours with my husband just holding me in bed. When I woke up, I felt like it was a nightmare until I realized that it had actually happened. I went into the bathroom and lifted up my shirt to look at my stomach. It actually felt like there was a hole going straight through me. I couldn't see it, but I could feel it there. I will never forget that feeling.

We were devastated. Now we had to break the news to everyone we had told. I felt ashamed. I was physically and emotionally drained. I couldn't even look at myself in the mirror most days. However, because we had told our family and friends, it was nice to have a close circle of support. I struggled over the next several months. It was hard to find joy in anything. This amazing dream that I had planned out never happened. Every time a milestone date came and went, there was just more disappointment.

Almost exactly a year from the day I found out I was pregnant the first time, I found out I was pregnant again. I was excited and scared. *Of course, miscarriages are common, right?* But surely, it won't happen to me again, right? Once that innocence was taken away from me, I couldn't help but worry about every little thing.

I saw the doctor around eight weeks along and, again, everything seemed normal. I scheduled an ultrasound for a few weeks later. We were pretty close on track with dates from our last pregnancy, and as the miscarriage anniversary date approached, I just wanted to get past it. It was August 26th, 2017. If I could make it past that date, then surely everything would be okay.

And then it started again. I started bleeding at a family gathering and immediately told my husband we needed to go home. I was almost eleven weeks pregnant. Everything happened so fast. I was at home in my bathroom this time. I couldn't believe it. It was August 26th, 2018. *Why? Why, on the same day a year apart?* I remember looking up at the sky the next morning thinking, *What did I ever do to deserve this?* I felt so ashamed, so let down by my body. I felt like I was letting my husband down. I felt completely alone. It was a very dark time for me. Most people who knew what I had been through told me how strong and resilient I was. But I didn't feel that way.

Knowing what I know now, I was strong. I was surviving.

After my second pregnancy loss, I made an appointment with my doctor to find out what was going wrong. He referred me to a reproductive endocrinologist. When he handed me the referral sheet, he had written Recurrent Pregnancy Loss as my diagnosis. My stomach dropped. *Could this happen to me again?* I was determined to achieve this dream of having our family. My husband and I decided to make the appointment with the specialist.

Ok, let's do this. It was a few days before Christmas. We went in for our appointment. I was feeling so nervous. *What if he tells me something I don't want to hear?* We didn't know what to expect. The doctor said we were going to be tested for a whole list of things: a full blood panel, genetic testing, sperm analysis, and internal ultrasounds. My head was spinning. I was determined to figure out whatever was causing my losses.

Everything was normal. The doctor found one small fibroid outside my uterus but said there was only a 5% chance that it was causing the miscarriages. That was good news to us! We went into this process positive, but still cautious. Our treatment plan was for me to take Letrozole with timed intercourse.

Boom! I was pregnant again. My husband was sleeping in bed and I woke him up with the positive pregnancy test. He had the biggest smile on his face; it was a look I will never forget. And all I could think was, *I hope I don't disappoint him again.* I was hopeful but scared after two losses. I called the RE office and they seemed shocked that I got pregnant on the first try. I went in for blood-work. My HCG levels did not rise appropriately and my progesterone dropped. I was put on progesterone suppositories.

When I went in for my six-week ultrasound, everything was measuring smaller than normal and there was no visible heartbeat. The doctor said it was simply too early to tell. I went back the next week and the sac and baby had grown a tiny bit. The doctor told us he was sorry but it wasn't going to be a viable pregnancy. Again, we were devastated. I was told I was going to need a D&C, I was relieved; miscarrying naturally the first two times was physically the hardest thing I have ever gone through. They told me it would be a few days until I would be able to get one. I was a nervous wreck. I just wanted to get it over with. It was unbearable to walk around knowing what I was carrying inside me. I felt like everyone that looked at me knew. I could barely function, but, somehow, I did. The specialist's office gave me the run-around for days and then finally scheduled me almost two weeks later.

The morning of the procedure, I went into the office for an ultrasound they told me was routine. When the nurse started the ultrasound, I was looking at the screen expecting to see what I had before. I saw the heartbeat and turned my head away and covered my eyes. I just remember saying, "What is that?" I knew what it was. OMG. She called the doctor in. The baby had grown to size and everything looked normal. I thought to myself, *This is my miracle baby.* I finally understood. I was still unable to feel positive at this point. I was in shock and excited at the same time.

I had to call my support system with the news. I felt like I had won the lottery. With no explanation, I was hopeful ... but I still had this reservation on my shoulders. We didn't know what would happen next.

I went to see my regular OB. He was shocked. After talking to him, and being over 11 weeks along, we thought we might be in the clear. Usually, at this point, it's not as common for women to lose the pregnancy as it is in the very early weeks. But it happened again. I just had that feeling. I went to the bathroom at work and wiped; it was bright red blood. *Here we go again.* I finished out the forty minutes left in my workday. The bleeding always happened fast in my case so I knew what to expect. Wanting some reassurance, I phoned the doctor. It was already happening. I thought to myself, *I can do this.* I could deliver my tiny baby at home in peace without anyone poking at me.

People who have had pregnancy losses know the pain. It's excruciating. And even though it's not a full-term baby, your body goes through the process. These are the things most people don't know. I understand why women are ashamed and quiet about the topic. It's a feeling you will never understand unless you've been there.

I swore to myself, *That's it.*

I'm finished passing everything. I've never had such an empty feeling. I now have to tell everyone again. It's the worst. I'm just wishing at this moment I could protect everyone from knowing this news. I'm wishing I never told anyone. It's just another heartbreak. Not only does it affect us, it affects our whole family. Pregnancy loss is an ugly thing. It's a grief that's different from any other. It's the loss of a life and the loss of your dreams for the future.

A week later, I was still cramping and bleeding. My lower back was killing me. I was worried that I hadn't passed everything on my own. Being farther along, it was physically much harder than I had previously experienced. I phoned the doctor and they had me go in for an ultrasound. Afterwards, the doctor told me I was just having reactionary contractions: everything was out of my uterus. It was a relief.

The pain was unreal. I had a follow-up with my doctor and he informed me that they saw some fibroids during my scan. He just told me to go home and heal up; then we could discuss further options. Later, I came to find out that I needed an open myomectomy to remove seven fibroids. The largest was the size of a grapefruit. All of this was news to me. After seeing the RE, he never diagnosed the fibroids as an issue. My OB was certain that was the only reason for our losses, given the size of the fibroid (which takes blood supply away from a growing fetus).

After I healed from the surgery, I was still certain that another pregnancy was not in the future for me. After discovering that my doctor believed the fibroids were the reason for our losses, we talked about it a lot. We considered adoption for a long time. *Was it worth it to put myself through that again? Was adoption right for us?* I have never felt so weak in my life, but at the same time I'd never felt stronger.

I made the sacrifice to give life. Anybody reading this who had to give a life back, you'll understand. It affects us in a different way. I often think that is why miscarriage and pregnancy loss is a topic that's taboo to talk about. It shouldn't be a shameful thing, but it feels that way. My hope for the future is that this changes. I often don't share my experiences, but I'm also not shy of talking about it.

I'm not really sure what the future holds. We are planning to try again. Recurrent pregnancy loss has changed my life in many ways. I've never felt so isolated in my life. It's not something that most people relate to. In fact, three consecutive miscarriages happen to only one percent of couples. Of course, I've had a great support system and multiple people to relate to. Being married for a few years now, we know the questions that are going to be asked at a social event: "Do you want kids?" "When are you having children?" And we come up with all these answers in our heads before we go somewhere. Because these are the questions people ask. It's reality. And it sucks.

I've struggled on and off over the past few years. I've struggled with depression and anxiety. I've struggled with loneliness and isolation. I've been in therapy for about a year now and it has helped tremendously. I'm proud of the progress I've made. One thing my miscarriages have taught me is how much of an optimist I am. Every person has their threshold of what they can allow themselves to go through. These have been some of the darkest times, but it helps to see a little light at the end of it all.

Public Figures Share Their Personal Experiences To Help Others

Kirstie Alley – *Three months. Unknown/Undisclosed.*

"When the baby was gone, I just didn't really get over it. Neither did my body.

"I so thoroughly convinced my body that it was still pregnant after nine months that I had milk coming from my breasts. I was still fat, I was still grieving, and I had just been told it was very possible I would never be able to have children. Fat, childless, with little hope for any future children ... that's when I began to get fat."

https://www.huffpost.com/entry/50-celebrities-who-opened-up-about-their-miscarriages_n_59de72a2e4b0fdad73b1b117

Public Figures Share Their Personal Experiences To Help Others

Meghan Markle – *(Believed to be) 12 weeks. Unknown/Undisclosed.*

The Losses We Share
By Meghan, The Duchess of Sussex

"It was a July morning that began as ordinarily as any other day: Make breakfast. Feed the dogs. Take vitamins. Find that missing sock. Pick up the rogue crayon that rolled under the table. Throw my hair in a ponytail before getting my son from his crib.

"After changing his diaper, I felt a sharp cramp. I dropped to the floor with him in my arms, humming a lullaby to keep us both calm, the cheerful tune a stark contrast to my sense that something was not right.

"I knew, as I clutched my firstborn child, that I was losing my second.

"Hours later, I lay in a hospital bed, holding my husband's hand. I felt the clamminess of his palm and kissed his knuckles, wet from both our tears. Staring at the cold white walls, my eyes glazed over. I tried to imagine how we'd heal.

"I recalled a moment last year when Harry and I were finishing up a long tour in South Africa. I was exhausted. I was breastfeeding our infant son, and I was trying to keep a brave face in the very public eye.

"'Are you OK?' a journalist asked me. I answered him honestly, not knowing that what I said would resonate with so many — new moms and older ones, and anyone who had, in their own way, been silently suffering. My off-the-cuff reply seemed to give people permission to speak their truth. But it wasn't responding honestly that helped me most, it was the question itself.

"'Thank you for asking,' I said. 'Not many people have asked if I'm OK.'

"Sitting in a hospital bed, watching my husband's heart break as he tried to hold the shattered pieces of mine, I realized that the only way to begin to heal is to first ask, 'Are you OK?'

"Are we? This year has brought so many of us to our breaking points. Loss and pain have plagued every one of us in 2020, in moments both fraught and debilitating. We've heard all the stories: A woman starts her day, as normal as any other, but then receives a call that she's lost her elderly mother to Covid-19. A man wakes feeling fine, maybe a little sluggish, but nothing out of the ordinary. He tests positive for the coronavirus and within weeks, he — like hundreds of thousands of others — has died.

"A young woman named Breonna Taylor goes to sleep, just as she's done every night before, but she doesn't live to see the morning because a police raid turns horribly wrong. George Floyd leaves a convenience store, not realizing he will take his last breath under the weight of someone's knee, and in his final moments, calls out for his mom. Peaceful protests become violent. Health rapidly shifts to sickness. In places where there was once community, there is now division.

"On top of all of this, it seems we no longer agree on what is true. We aren't just fighting over our opinions of facts; we are polarized over whether the fact is, in fact, a fact. We are at odds over whether science is real. We are at odds over whether an election has been won or lost. We are at odds over the value of compromise.

"That polarization, coupled with the social isolation required to fight this pandemic, has left us feeling more alone than ever.

"When I was in my late teens, I sat in the back of a taxi zipping through the busyness and bustle of Manhattan. I looked out the window and saw a woman on her phone in a flood of tears. She was standing on the sidewalk, living out a private moment very publicly. At the time, the city was new to me, and I asked the driver if we should stop to see if the woman needed help.

"He explained that New Yorkers live out their personal lives in public spaces. 'We love in the city, we cry in the street, our emotions and stories there for anybody to see,' I remember him telling me. 'Don't worry, somebody on that corner will ask her if she's OK.'

"Now, all these years later, in isolation and lockdown, grieving the loss of a child, the loss of my country's shared belief in what's true, I think of that woman in New York. What if no one stopped? What if no one saw her suffering? What if no one helped?

"I wish I could go back and ask my cabdriver to pull over. This, I realize, is the danger of siloed living — where moments sad, scary or sacrosanct are all lived out alone. There is no one stopping to ask, 'Are you OK?'

"Losing a child means carrying an almost unbearable grief, experienced by many but talked about by few. In the pain of our loss, my husband and I discovered that in a room of 100 women, 10 to 20 of them will have suffered from miscarriage. Yet despite the staggering commonality of this pain, the conversation remains taboo, riddled with (unwarranted) shame, and perpetuating a cycle of solitary mourning.

"Some have bravely shared their stories; they have opened the door, knowing that when one person speaks truth, it gives license for all of us to do the same. We have learned that when people ask how any of us are doing, and when they really listen to the answer, with an open heart and mind, the load of grief often becomes lighter — for all of us. In being invited to share our pain, together we take the first steps toward healing.

"So this Thanksgiving, as we plan for a holiday unlike any before — many of us separated from our loved ones, alone, sick, scared, divided and perhaps struggling to find something, anything, to be grateful for — let us commit to asking others, 'Are you OK?' As much as we may disagree, as physically distanced as we may be, the truth is that we are more connected than ever because of all we have individually and collectively endured this year.

"We are adjusting to a new normal where faces are concealed by masks, but it's forcing us to look into one another's eyes — sometimes filled with warmth, other times with tears. For the first time, in a long time, as human beings, we are really seeing one another.

"Are we OK?

"We will be."

A version of this article appears in print on Nov. 25, 2020, Section A, Page 23 of the New York edition with the headline: The Losses We Share. https://www.nytimes.com/2020/11/25/opinion/meghan-markle-miscarriage.html

Public Figures Share Their Personal Experiences To Help Others

Tori Amos – *3 months. Unknown/Undisclosed.*

"[The song]'Spark' is about when I miscarried in 1996. I was three months pregnant and very excited. All of a sudden I woke up one morning and started to feel bad. The songs started coming soon after. I was really angry at God.

"Once you've felt life in your body, you can't go back to having been a woman that's never carried life. The other thing is feeling something dying inside you and you're still alive. Obviously when it was happening, it was already over, but in my mind, you don't know that it's over yet.

"There's nothing you can do, so you surrender and then... start again."

https://www.songfacts.com/facts/tori-amos/spark

"I went through a lot of different feelings after the miscarriage -- you go through everything possible. You question what is fair, you get angry with the spirit for not wanting to come, you keep asking why. And then, as I was going through the anger and the sorrow and the why, the songs started to come. going through the anger and the sorrow and the why, the songs started to come. Before I was even aware, they were coming to me in droves. Looking back, that's the way it's always happened for me in my life. When things get really empty for me -- empty in my outer life -- in my inner life, the music world, the songs come across galaxis to find me.

"People had a very hard time talking to me about what had happened, and I had a hard time talking about it. But the songs seemed to have such an easy time talking to me. And I began to feel the freedom of the music.

"Each song would show me a certain side of herself because of what I was going through. So a song like 'cruel' came to me out of my anger. 'She's your cocaine' and 'iieee' came out of a sense of loss and sacrifice. And other songs celebrated the fact that I had found a new appreciation for life through this loss.

[...]"There's a deep love on this record ['From the Choirgirl Hotel']. This is not a victim's record. It deals with sadness, but it's a passionate record -- passionate for life, for the life force. And a respect for the miracle of life."

http://www.yessaid.com/pr_1998-05_choirgirl-promobio.html

16

Nathalia's Purpose

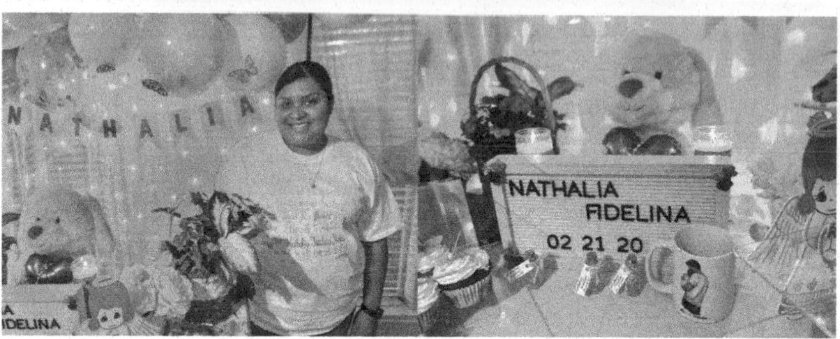

by Dina Mejia

The first place I went to in my mind, while holding my lifeless child in my arms, was the day I last saw her alive: my last ultrasound, when I could hear the echoing of her heartbeat. All I could hear was my dear Nathalia's heartbeat. *Why?! Why her?! Why me?!*

August 2, 2017

I receive a phone call giving me my diagnosis, "Unfortunately, you have Polycystic Ovary Syndrome," (also known as PCOS). It explains why I have irregular cycles and weight gain. I was so devastated, my heart broke into pieces. Being engaged to my high school sweetheart (whom I've been dating for six years now), we were getting ready to start our family in just two more months. Then I get this news, "You may struggle with infertility and may not be able to hold a child full term."

So many mixed emotions went through my mind and I could not help but think maybe I should never marry. My husband deserves to have a family of his own. *What if I could never make him a father? What if he sees me as less than a woman? What if he leaves me for someone else? What if he lives a double life?* All of these scenarios just kept replaying in my mind. My head was spinning.

I learned as a child how to snap out of things when I feel "Satan" put his arm around me and try to manipulate my thoughts. I've struggled with anxiety, depression, and panic attacks all of my life. The devil wants me. Suicidal thoughts have always haunted me. Learning to be able to fight the demons is like having super powers.

God is the one and only who will get us through anything! We must learn how to let him in. Many would ask, "If He is so Great, then why do bad things happen?" He gives us a chance to make our own mistakes and learn on our own. Without Him, I would not be here. He brought my husband to me during in the darkest part of my life.

I was just thinking of ways to tell my husband I could not marry him. I was embarrassed that I may not be able to do the one thing we, as women, are meant to live for. A couple of weeks later, I told him. He said to me, "Babes, marriage is about being together for better or worse. I Love you and I want to marry you. We can start trying now; doctors are not always right. God will give us a miracle. We just have to have faith."

Well, here we are, three years later.

November 2019:

My mother's best friend of almost forty years suffered a stroke. She passed away on November 24th. She was in the ICU for three days. She was a wonderful, strong Christian lady that knew the word of God like the palms of her hands. Before and after our work shifts, I went with my mother to be with her for those three days until her family made the decision to let her go. It was hard seeing her body for the last time and knowing I would never hear her laughter, her prayers, her cries; and never again taste her delicious lemon pies. For the very last time, I touched her feet. She had a perfect pedicure with beautiful, fall-colored nail polish. As I moved up to hold her hand and gave her a goodbye kiss on her forehead, I whispered into her ear how much I loved her and how I was going to miss her so dearly.

The day before, I watched a nurse come in and check her oxygen tube. She opened her eyes. I saw her open her eyes. I felt so much hope. I came back home and got the call at exactly four a.m. She's gone. FOREVER. Well, I had never experienced anything like that before. It was cold, sad, dark, as if the world just stopped moving, then silence. All the memories I had growing up with her just came flooding back, so many details. I know now that that is this reality, this is it: the cycle of life.

November 26, 2019

It is now the day for the viewing. As I walk in to see our dear, beloved friend, I get this cold but also warm feel to my skin. I see her lying there, lifeless, no blood flowing through her veins; it is clear, SHE IS GONE. I try very hard to keep being strong for my mom and the rest of the family. We sit and the ceremony goes on.

The ceremony over, my mother, sister, and I go to the restroom. I proceed to put water on my face to help refresh myself. After, I go into the stall and see some blood on my underwear. I have irregular cycles; I have not had a cycle in about four to five months now. We get home. I take a shower, put a pad on, and watch a little TV after the very long, emotionally exhausting day. I am not looking forward to tomorrow's burial.

NOVEMBER 27, 2019

I wake up. There's no blood at all on my pad. That was no surprise; that was normal to for me. Irregular cycles are very stressful; you get false hopes.

It's now time to get ready for the burial. There is no point in wearing a pad if there isn't any blood. When we arrive at the cemetery, I feel wetness in my underwear. There are not restrooms near us; I will have to wait until we get to the family's after-gathering. Upon our arrival at the reception, I quickly check and there's a small amount of spotting again. I quickly change, then go and help the host.

NOVEMBER 30, 2019

My sister finds out she is indeed pregnant. It is her sixth pregnancy after three miscarriages. I am a bit envious, but excited to be an aunt again. It feels so fast, like a slap in the face. I have been trying to conceive for three years with no luck and here she is, not trying at all.

DECEMBER 20, 2019

I work as a bus attendant for students with special needs. One of my students, who is in a wheelchair, always carries snacks on the side of their backpack. I am not a fan of Cheetos at all. *Why did I feel the urge to cry because of how desperate I was to have those Cheetos at six A.M.? Only someone who is out of their mind would eat junk food for breakfast!* Well, call me crazy, because as soon as I finished the first half of my shift, I rushed to the grocery store and bought a huge bag for breakfast!

CHRISTMAS EVE 2019

Now that I try to remember what exactly drove me to take a pregnancy test, I cannot seem to remember. I have many pregnancy tests under my sink, so I took a test first thing in the morning. When I looked at the test, I thought to myself, *Too good to be true; this is what I want to see. It's not real.* There was a very, very faint, positive line. That pregnancy test did not convince me at all.

It was time for me to prep to go to my sister's house for the holiday. (In my Hispanic community, we celebrate Christmas on Christmas Eve and on Christmas Day.) At my sister's house, tragedy occurs: my sister has to go to the hospital and will not be celebrating Christmas. She was pregnant for six weeks with twins. Unfortunately, she loses both twins. There goes our Christmas.

December 27, 2019

I decide to take another pregnancy test. Again, I have no idea what draws me to take another test. There aren't a good amount of symptoms that make me believe that I am pregnant this time. Even though I got a very faint positive test last time, I highly doubt I am pregnant. Well, SURPRISE! It is a VERY DARK, FULL, DYE-STEALER POSITIVE!! I'm over the moon with joy and cannot believe what I am seeing! My husband is just on the other side of our bathroom door. I tell him, "BABE, I THINK I AM PREGNANT." So, he looks at the test and the look in his eyes says it all. He is emotionally excited and says, "WE DID IT; YOU'RE PREGNANT. WE ARE GOING TO BE PARENTS!" He touches and kisses me, and our little, tiny baby.

I called many places to look for an OBGYN that would accept my insurance. Since I found out I was pregnant on a Friday, the only place that was open on a Saturday was a primary doctor. So, I took the appointment because they would just draw my blood to confirm if I was for-sure pregnant.

December 28, 2019

It's time for the doctor's appointment! I did not get much sleep the night before because I was so excited and anxious to confirm this pregnancy. I felt this joy in my heart. This motivation for life was the greatest feeling ever. My husband decided to take the day off of work to accompany me to this appointment. We have arrived at our destination. I checked in and we waited to be called. When they called out my name, I felt this nervous but excited feeling.

The doctor was very rude; she did not acknowledge my husband at all, did not greet either one us. She just asked, "What brings you in today? I see you believe you may be pregnant?" I answered, "Yes, I have PCOS, irregular cycles. I am not sure when I had my last cycle to be exact; it's been between four and five months. We have been trying to conceive for three years now. I have not been feeling too well. I've been much more tired than usual, my lower back is hurting so much, I feel bloated, and I am spotting as we speak, and I have been for almost a month now; it comes and goes, and I am having pains in my left pelvic area." Her response was,

"Sounds to me like you're having an ectopic pregnancy because everything you're telling me is not normal. We don't have an ultrasound machine here, but I suggest you go and get it out now. Just go to the E.R. and tell them you have an ectopic pregnancy and you need to get it removed as soon as possible. This is deadly; you could be dying soon!"

To begin with, this lady did not check anything on me; she only pressed down where I told her it hurt and I told her that I did not feel comfortable with her pressing on me like that. I could not help but cry because of what she had just said to us. She killed our joy. She spoke like nothing mattered. She said, "Don't cry; it might not even have a heartbeat." As soon as a child is conceived, no matter how big or how small, IT MATTERS, DAMNIT!!!

My husband hugged me and took me to the E.R. and there, we told the kind nurse what was going on. The hospital staff was so kind, so sweet to us. I was taken to an ultrasound room and got an ultrasound done. About an hour later, the doctor walked in and told us, "Congratulations, mommy and daddy; you're having a baby! You are five weeks! I want you to come back in two days to get your HCG levels checked to make sure your baby is growing the way it should be. In the meantime, look for an OBGYN to keep checking on you. I will see you in two days. Again, CONGRATULATIONS."

My mother lives with us. As soon as we got home, I couldn't help but tell her. She was excited for us, especially because she knew of my troubles. Two days later, I went to get my HCG levels checked and they were perfect! Baby was growing and the doctor said the spotting could be normal, as some pregnant women with PCOS make it to full term with no problems.

December 30, 2019

My OBGYN appointment is with one of the worst doctors ever! This damn lady literally stuck the transvaginal ultrasound wand in very roughly, as if she was rushing. She said, "I'm sorry, but there's no hope here; your body is disposing of this on it's own. So whatever comes out, put it in this urine sample cup and bring it to me. You don't even get your period. I only see a yolk sac, nothing more." I understand that this is normal for her; it does not matter, but I don't experience this every day! She did not do any blood work or anything. If I would have known a little more about pregnancy, maybe my daughter would be here now.

Some days, I feel like I failed her. Would I have been one sorry-ass mom who couldn't protect her in my womb, much less in the real world? I ask myself that all the time, but I am no doctor. They are doctors for a reason: they are the ones who needed to know how to help take care of me and my pregnancy – that's what they got their medical degree for. It's their specialty not mine. It's sad that it had to get this far for me to get my head straight. I wish I'd had more knowledge and would have had enough courage then to do more for myself and for my child. I will forever feel this way.

So, I did not get any type of blood work that day. All I felt was helpless. The doctor didn't even bother to ask for a follow-up to see how my pregnancy was going to develop. Right away, I began searching for other doctors that would accept my insurance, but no luck. I know now that it shouldn't have been be so hard to find a good doctor that was willing to provide the care I needed. This was now the third doctor I had been to but no one was helping me. It was nothing but negative comments on how unviable my pregnancy was. How was I supposed to stay positive and hopeful? The only thing that kept me going was my husband and my mother.

The minute my husband saw the test, he would not stop talking to our little poppy seed. Since that moment on, he would whisper to our baby every day before leaving for work, *I love you baby. Keep growing strong.* He'd give me my kiss and I was so much more motivated to work to provide for our baby.

On our way home from that horrible experience with the last OBGYN, my husband and I were still excited to announce our miracle news to our families. Yes, it was very early on in my pregnancy, but we thought about what the doctor from a few days ago had told us, about how far I was and that the baby was growing the way it was suppose to. He seemed very positive about everything and suggested I get a follow-up with an OBGYN to confirm my last cycle and how big the fetus should be. We made the crazy decision to announce to our families on New Year's!

December 31, 2019

It is now New Year's Eve! A few more hours until we make the announcement. We were debating announcing now or waiting further. Since my sister had a miscarriage a few days ago I do not want this to affect her and make her feel like I am not taking her feelings into consideration. I am, of course, but I think to myself that I have always been supportive and been there for her on her worst days, and also on her best. I've pushed my feelings to the side and been happy for her. I think she'll do the same for me since she knows my condition and how long I have been waiting for this day.

I gain the courage to speak to her privately and tell her how much I feel for her loss. As I tell her privately, she is not as happy for me as I had hoped but I completely understand. Maybe it was selfish of me to say anything, but I had to. My happiness counts too and I need to make the best of it in the best possible ways. I ask my sister if it is okay for me to announce my pregnancy to the rest of the family at midnight; I wanted her very honest opinion about it. She says that it is okay and that she's happy for me even if it doesn't seem that way.

We hugged, we cried, and spoke about how we would have had children the same age. It was a great conversation. I was sad for her, but excited about my baby. It may sound selfish, but I was so happy. I had been waiting for this miracle for years now, and it was finally my time. I have five siblings and I am the only one with no living children. I've never wanted anything more than to experience motherhood and all the challenges that come with it.

I currently have a sister-in-law who is pregnant with her second child. She is 33 years old and has had many weight loss surgeries. We've had our differences, but she is the type of person who loves the spotlight and feels she knows best about anything.... Well that story is for another time. She wanted to leave soon, so I told her about my pregnancy right before she left. My other brother, who is her husband, was working at the time. I did not want him to find out from anyone but me. I kindly asked her not to say anything to him. This lady was not happy for me at all. She looked at me from head to toe and said, "Congrats," with no feel to it at all. Her pregnancy announcements have always been exciting and I am always the first to jump up and hug her. It tells a lot about a person when they react a certain way about the most sensitive part in someone's life. It is what it is; what can I do? We can't meet everyone's expectations.

My family and I began to play charades; the time to make our announcement was near! I had bought a small chalkboard from Hobby Lobby and written "SURPRISE! BABY MEJIA COMING 2020!" on it. When it was my husband's turn to play, I held the charades board and had my chalkboard behind it. My husband held the microphone we were using and said, "I'M PREGNANT!" My family was like, "Huh? Wait! WHAT?! OH MY GOODNESS!!! YAYYYYY!!! CONGRATULATIONS!!!!!!!!" They hugged us and gave us kisses and best wishes. Since that day on, everyone would go to my belly and show it so much love and affection. God, do I miss those moments every day.

After midnight, my husband and I left to see his family and give them the news. Long story short, his family and I were not on very good speaking terms at the time. When we arrived, I did not even have the opportunity to use my board to make the announcement. Everyone was scattered around and didn't respect the fact that we needed everyone together in order to give them the news. So, we just told his mother (whom I've had some issues with). I showed her the board and all she said was, "I hope it"s a boy; I don't want another granddaughter. I want a grandson!"

Her reaction was as I expected; it's no surprise that that was her response. But all I could do was just walk outside and stand and look at the fireworks and keep myself from crying. I don't know if maybe I overreacted, but I took what she said to heart. I had really hoped for her response to be, "CONGRATULATIONS! I KNOW HOW LONG YOU'VE BEEN WAITING FOR THIS MOMENT! WE ALL HAVE! WHATEVER GOD GIVES US, WE ARE BLESSED!" Instead, my heart broke. I'd wished this pregnancy would have changed her way of seeing me. I guess, in a way, I'd expected her to treat me like a person, but no, nothing had changed. Yes, many would say that my husband needs to stick up for me. He has many times, but his mom is just very judgmental and nothing is ever good enough for her. In the beginning, we did get along very well, but we had a disagreement about some situation about two years before I got pregnant, and it changed our relationship completely.

Ever since that pregnancy announcement, I've kept my distance even more and so has my husband, for my wellbeing and our baby. It had already been quite a year; I did not need any more stress coming my way, especially if it was not necessary. Just my job itself was mentally stressful. I apologize if this is way too much information, but this is what happened during my pregnancy. This is what maybe caused my miscarriage: STRESS.

January 25, 2019

The bleeding continued like a period. There was no pain, no cramps, no blood clots, but my lower back ached, I was always nauseated, and I would always vomit. These symptoms, for some reason, would get worse on Fridays. I had to spend time in the E.R. The doctor came in and ruled my pregnancy a "Threatening Miscarriage." Well, that was a huge blow. The drive home was so quiet. I cried, but quickly tried to keep my head up and to continue being strong for the both of us.

The following week, I called in sick because I was bleeding and really just wanted to be in bed. Later in the week, I went to my first official doctor's appointment to get this baby checked and guess what? There was a heartbeat! 178bpm My baby had a strong heartbeat! This doctor was amazing, such a sweet lady. She said, "As of now, your baby is great; it has a strong heartbeat. But there is something I am worried about: you have a subchorionic hematoma. That is what is causing your bleeding. Most of the time, it will taper off as the baby grows. We will keep monitoring this. I suggest you take it easy and I want to see you again in a week from now to see if this has grown. Congratulations! Here are your pictures and I will see you in a week."

The following week came and the damn subchorionic hematoma had grown. The doctor put me on bed rest for two weeks.

February 14, 2020 Valentine's Day

Time for my checkup again and well, I was very anxious and nervous to see my baby. When I walked out of my home to get in my truck, I got a surprise. It was my husband; he wanted to see our baby so he got out of work early to accompany me to the appointment. This was his first time coming with me to this doctor and the doctor congratulated him and shook his hand. I really appreciated her acknowledging my husband. The doctor proceeded to do the ultrasound and there was our Nathalia! A lot bigger than last time with a strong heartbeat. Her Daddy spoke to her, and she MOVED! She played with her tiny little hands and was clapping! She kicked! I could not believe my eyes; I could not believe that there was a tiny human growing in my belly and she recognized daddy's voice. I was so excited, I wanted to take the ultrasound machine home with me to keep an eye on my baby at all times, but I didn't. Oh, how I miss her.

Well, the damn subchorionic hematoma was growing. At that point, I did not know what to think anymore. I had to accept whatever God's Will was going to be, had to be. I had to hope for the best and prepare for the worst. The doctor wanted to see me again the following week. Hubby and I looked forward for my nephew's birthday dinner that night. It would keep our minds off of things for a while with a little distraction.

February 19, 2020

Today is my next appointment to check my baby. My doctor suggests I get blood drawn to check if I'm immune to Rubella, as well as other lab tests. Also, she asks if I want to get a genetic test done since I have two nieces with Down syndrome. She wants to make sure there are no chromosomal abnormalities. My husband and I are in love with our little baby; we want this baby more than anything, with or without chromosomal abnormalities. We accepted the test either way as those tests will be giving us the gender of our baby.

My bleeding was not getting any lighter, so I was referred to a high-risk specialist. I called as soon as I got home to schedule an appointment for the following week. My appointment was set for February 26th. I was anxiously waiting for the appointment; I would not go back to work until I got the all clear to return from this high-risk specialist.

February 20, 2020

This day, I got upset; three people made me so angry. Already knowing this was a high-risk pregnancy, you'd think my family would have had some consideration. I regret it. I regret not putting myself before others. I should have been selfish. I took a nice warm shower to help me relax a little.

One hour later, I felt wetness in my underwear. I went to the bathroom and saw that my pad was full of plain water, no spotting, just water. I called the on-call nurse and told her everything that was going on to see if I needed to go to the hospital. She asked if it was a lot and I said, "Yes, but it has not continued. There was maybe a good handful of it." She told me to go to the E.R. and so I did. The doctor quickly took me back and used the ultrasound on my belly. HEARTBEAT. There she was, fighting. She was a fighter. She wasn't giving up. I felt a huge sense of relief.

FEBRUARY 21, 2020

Hubby and I decided to take a nap around six pm. My mother got off of work that day at eight o'clock. We woke up around 7:45 pm and my husband left to go get my mom. About 10 minutes after he left, I went to the bathroom. I peed, and well, since the spotting had always been there, in a way it was normal, but at the same time, I wanted it to go away. I wanted it to stop and to leave me the hell alone. Damn subchorionic hematoma. Then, when I stood up, I heard this gush sound between my legs. I put my hand on my lower area. There she was: MY BABY!

My chest felt so heavy it literally hurt. My body was numb. I was in shock. I couldn't believe it; I didn't want to believe it. This was not happening, not to me. I fell to my knees, holding my lifeless child. I know I may sound crazy but I thought maybe with CPR I could bring her back. I want her back. All I could do was scream. It was silent. I could not hear myself scream. *Did I scream? Was this going on in my head? I want my baby!! Please, god, give her back!!!* I was so alone. No one was home.

I was angry, but at the same time I was not. I was angry at the fact that I wasn't gone with her. I was angry that I was still here and she wasn't. I was angry that this joy took so many years for me to have, but then it was taken away so quickly. I was angry at myself for not being strong enough to keep her inside of me. I was angry at my husband. I was angry at my family. In that moment, I wanted to die. I wanted to disappear.

Then I see my husband come in. He tries to pick me up. He's talking, but I can't hear a word he's saying. I remember him running out. I held my baby. I held her. I looked at every single detail: her feet, her second toe was long like mine; her left hand was over her chest; her legs were crossed together. When I looked at her stomach, I saw that her intestines were out. I'm not sure what that means. I wish I knew the answer to all of my questions, but I don't. I do battle with this to this day. As long as I live, I will forever wonder why. *Why, damnit? Why?!*

My mom came in. She grabbed my baby and held her. She hugged me and said things, but I did not hear anything. It sounded like when you've fallen in the water and you hear a far distance echoing. It's blank. I do not remember how I got to my bed. I do not remember getting dressed. I remember nothing. My daughter never saw the light of day, she never breathed this oxygen, and she passed with no sin. I know exactly where she is.

My brother and both sisters came to see me, and took me to the E.R. I had refused to go because I was afraid for some reason. I'm not sure why, but I was. There was nothing more that could have been done. I was aggressive; I came in the hospital screaming and crying out loud. It was the loudest I have ever cried. They asked if I wanted them to take my baby. I said, "HELL NO, FOR WHAT? SO Y'ALL CAN MESS WITH HER? TO CUT HER IN PIECES AND CHECK FOR ABNORMALITIES. NO THANK YOU!" They said, "Do you want to keep her, or do you want us to take care of it? We'll throw her in the hazardous container and burn her with the rest of the trash. If not, we could also bury her with other remains we dispose of." If my family had not been there, I think I may have really lost it. It was absolutely inappropriate. They let me go home; the entire way, I cried and cried like there was no tomorrow.

February 22, 2020

No sleep, non-stop crying, and still, no bleeding. We lit candles around my baby and prayed for her. My father and mother-in-law came over in the morning to pay their respects. I did not feel that my mother-in-law was sincere at all about how sorry she was for me losing my child. (She will never know that my baby was a girl: she didn't love her from the beginning. She doesn't love her now. She doesn't deserve to know.) My father-in-law was the sweetest: he held me and rubbed my head and cried with me. He said the sweetest things to me and gave me exactly the comfort I needed.

I feel this urge to vomit. I still have my symptoms. Sadly, I still have morning sickness. I come back from the restroom and see that my in-laws are no longer in my room. They were not welcome to see my baby. My Nathalia was already prepared to be laid to rest; she was wrapped up in a blanket. Why in the world was my mother-in-law unwrapping her and shining a flashlight all over my baby's face? RUDE! In this moment, I was certainly not in the mood to give her any type of attention. She left.

February 23, 2020

It was a Sunday; I decided to go to church. As I sat there, praying for strength and asking God to keep my child, to hold her and to let her know how much I love her, I felt this huge gush of blood go down both of my legs. I was bleeding, three days after losing my baby, but still, I felt no pain. After that moment, there was no more bleeding, still no pain, and no cramping. The following Thursday, I started feeling what I believe were contractions. I was in pain for about a month after that. I was so depressed I had no appetite, nothing.

March 18, 2020

Happy birthday to me. I prayed to God, years back, and made a birthday wish to be pregnant or be a mother by my 25th birthday. Well, there goes my birthday wish. All I want is to be a mom to a living child.

May 2020

Mother's day is here. My husband gives me not one but TWO puppies (two dachshunds: Milo and Minnie)! I love them so dearly. This does not change the fact that I still want my Babygirl, but it is comforting and does help me get through my days.

September 2, 2020

Today was supposed to be my due date. Now, I know a small percentage of babies are actually born on their due dates, but this makes me feel like I should be preparing to be coming home with a baby by now. There should be a crib in my room, but there isn't. This is something I will forever do battle with. I will continue learning how to live without her.

I will keep my promises. I will continue living. I will not lose myself. I will continue laughing and smiling.

I LOVE YOU, NATHALIA FIDELINA MEJIA HERNANDEZ, February 21, 2020. You are missed.

Public Figures Share Their Personal Experiences To Help Others

Celine Dion – *Miscarriage. Unknown/Undisclosed.*

"It's life, you know? A lot of people go through this. We tried four times to have a child. We're still trying."

https://www.huffpost.com/entry/21-celebrities-who-opened-up-about-their-miscarriages-to-support-other-women_n_563104aee4b0c66bae5a817d

"I thought as long as my health permitted me and unless my doctor thought physically I couldn't do it, then I would go on with the IVF until someone told me to stop.

"We didn't want to feel like we were playing yo-yo—I'm pregnant. I'm not pregnant. I'm pregnant. I'm not pregnant—so we didn't want to do this thing. But we did have a miscarriage.

"I will be the happiest one to tell you when I'm pregnant. And if not, I'm the luckiest artist, especially wife and mother of a wonderful son. So I'm glad."

https://www.infertilityaide.com/celebrities/celine-dions-infertility-struggle-7-ivf-cycles

17

Quarantine Losses

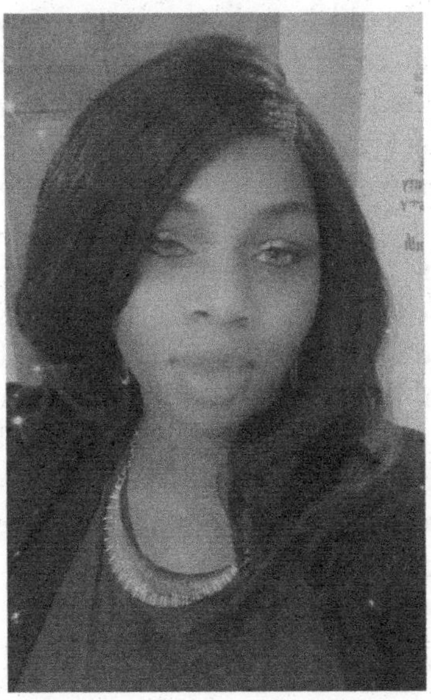

by Ms. Khat-Eyes

I thought because of my age (36) and the fact that I had not conceived to date, that I wasn't meant to be a mother or maybe that was not God's plan for me. But then came my favorite guy, with what I called "Super-Sperm," who got me pregnant the first week of Covid quarantine in Michigan.

We waited some time before telling people. I initially wanted to wait until at least 20 weeks, based on what I've read and watched on YouTube. But although I was labeled high risk, after my first ultrasound, the doctor and ultrasound tech reassured me that I wasn't showing any signs of miscarriage. So reluctantly, we started letting the dog (I'm a dog mom!) out of the bag. I had some spotting and bleeding, but it was waved off as a regular occurrence during first trimester.

The last time I bled before a doctor visit, I was twelve weeks. That day, I had a small amount of blood-spotting for a short time and then it went away. I didn't think anything of it because I was told multiple times that it was normal. That must have been Baby Sparks' final warning sign.

The next week, at my 13-week follow-up, they were initially not planning to do an ultrasound, only a Doppler heartbeat check. But I insisted. They did the Doppler, but could not find the heartbeat. So, the doctor grabbed the small portable ultrasound cart. She found the baby, but did not see a heartbeat. Then she did a vaginal ultrasound; still no movement. She finally said, "Unfortunately guys, I hate to say this, but there is no heartbeat. I've looked and don't see any movement or sign of life!"

They then used the big ultrasound machine to take measurements and see if there was anything visible that could have changed. We were told that although I should have been about 13 weeks and 5 days, the baby was measuring at 10 weeks. Outside of the small amount of blood the previous week, I had seen no sign that there was something wrong. I immediately felt every emotion my body could, all at once. I felt even more ashamed and embarrassed, like I accidentally farted in a room full of people.

I ended up having a sectional D&C because the sac was still inside and intact. I felt so lost, hurt, ashamed, embarrassed, like a failure. It's been a week since the D&C and I still catch myself rubbing or grabbing my stomach out of habit. My body is still bloated and giving me pregnancy cravings. I wrote a note back on May 1 to my unborn about my hopes and fears for raising him/her and just last night, I wrote another one to my angel baby! I plan to print both out and put them in a memory box I started for my angel baby boy!

Public Figures Share Their Personal Experiences To Help Others

Tamar Braxton – *Miscarriage. Unknown/Undisclosed.*

"I'm very nervous about going through that whole process of IVF again, because having a loss after going through it is really devastating. It really is a loss you can't explain.

"Early on, there was a time where I was like, 'I don't want kids! I'm all about my career,' and my gynecologist said, 'Here's the thing, Tamar: You never know what life is ever going to throw you, so you should really consider freezing your eggs.' Vince and I talked about it, and when I went for my initial IVF—when I was just going to freeze my eggs—I didn't know that I had infertility issues. I was blocked on both sides as if I had my tubes tied. I was 34 when I found this out. They don't know what causes that. The devil? Ha! It's just my makeup. The doctors didn't think I couldn't have kids; it wasn't going to happen [the natural] way. I didn't even know that until I went to go freeze my eggs. But I was cool with it, because at that time I didn't even want to have kids. Now, I would have started at 28, 29, 30, but you don't know until you know.

"What happened was, right after IVF, coincidentally I got pregnant with Logan. He's the best thing that ever happened to Vince and I. Considering I was told I probably wouldn't be able to have kids [without help], that's why Logan is a real miracle baby.

"At first, right after I had him, I'm like, 'I'm not having any more kids!' I hated being pregnant! I wanted an apple martini the whole time. I craved it. [Pregnancy] was hell. And then you fall in love with this kid—this crazy miracle—and all of the sudden want more. He has enriched my life so much.

"Vince and I started trying for a second child, but it just didn't work. My gynecologist was like, 'You need to use the eggs you were able to freeze.' I didn't want to go through the whole IVF situation again because I knew what [was involved]. My personality changed. I was a hateful heffer. And I didn't want to be hateful! I knew what it did. And I was so hungry! I ate all day! But I knew I wanted a baby more than I cared about all these other things. So, me and Vince went through getting the injections all over again to get my uterus ready to have the embryo implanted. And when you're 38 or 39, the doctors only want to implant one embryo. I had six viable embryos, and four were healthy. But when you're in your late 30s, the doctors only want to implant one at a time because there's a higher percentage rate of multiple births. Knowing that they could only implant one at at time was devastating to me. Because if that one didn't stick, I knew I would have to go through the entire process again. Aside from the physical toll on your body from all the shots, the IV's, the blood work, etc., it's so expensive to keep going through it. No matter how much money people think you have, expensive is expensive! And there's no guarantee it's going to work.

"I got the implantation, and I went for my pregnancy test, and it was positive. Three days later though, they called to tell me my numbers were going down. When your numbers are going down, it's a wrap. I wasn't pregnant that long after my pregnancy test.

"I didn't know how I was going to get out of my bed for a couple weeks. But you just do, you know? The same choice you make to be courageous and go through this process is the same choice to get up and keep going. It was hard because I still had to work. But after the miscarriage, I wanted so badly for the other things in my life to work. My tour got canceled. Of course everybody knows what happened at [The Real]. My album came out and I couldn't support it. I had to stop *Dancing with the Stars*. I just wanted to feel like I achieved something that I set out to do. When it didn't happen, I felt like I was going to have an emotional breakdown. It was tough.

"But I refuse any more losses. I feel like I deserve wins. I'm not going to take anything less than that. Like the music I'm getting ready to put out—it's a 'W' for me because I feel like it's amazing. And I'm proud of it. And if I decide to go through this whole situation again with the IVF, then that's a 'W' for me, because it's hard to make that decision for me. So I won! I've dedicated myself to losing the weight from IVF too, because it won't come off until it's ready. So being comfortable with that? That's a win for me.

"But this is still a struggle. And sometimes when I'm alone, I feel less than a woman. Like a failure. And it's very sensitive and it's very hard to talk about and you don't want to share it with a lot of people when you're going through it. Vince and I didn't discuss it with anyone. I didn't even tell my mom because you feel like if you tell somebody it's bad luck. I just wish people would be more sensitive and maybe ask 'How can I help you? Is there anything I can do?'

"But when someone hasn't gone through it, they don't understand the level of the loss. You don't want to hear, 'Oh, it will all work out. Don't worry.' Like, 'how do you know?' People that say, 'Oh, you can always adopt,' drives me crazy. I think adoption is great, but I want to have my own baby. I have these embryos in the freezer, and I want to be able to see what they look like. Are they anything like Logan? I put myself through that situation because I want to see that outcome. I can't lie and tell you at this point Vince and I have not talked about adoption or a surrogacy, but if I can have my own, of course [I want to].

"I tell my girlfriends, 'will you please go freeze your eggs?' Everyone is waiting for the right guy and the right time and the right financial block that they're in, but we kind of take it for granted that we'll always be able to have children. Go and do it. Because you never know. Once you turn 35, they view that as a high-risk pregnancy.

"But just know that making the decision to freeze your eggs is just the start. You have to find the right doctor and fertility center. I went to two different places originally. The doctor that we went with said, 'we want quality, not quantity.' That stuck with me. And know that you can't be on the hustle and bustle when going through the egg-freezing process. You have to be really committed to it because you basically live at the doctor's office. You have to go there almost daily for an ultrasound and bloodwork. Every day is something else. Vince and a nurse did the shots for me. I'm a real wimp. You also have to disrupt your day because you have to take these shots on time, and the older you get, the more strict your doctors are about the time that you take it. You'll sometimes even get depressed during this. You're like, 'I did this to myself?!' You're bruised and you look six months pregnant and you're hungry all the time. But you always have to remember why you're doing this. You do it because you want to have the final result.

"Logan is such a blessing. He's like my best friend. But I know that I have the gift of responsibility to be the woman that he has to look up to. And I will not fail at that."

https://www.glamour.com/story/tamar-braxton-opens-up-about-her-recent-miscarriage-after-ivf

18

Remember Me, Rain

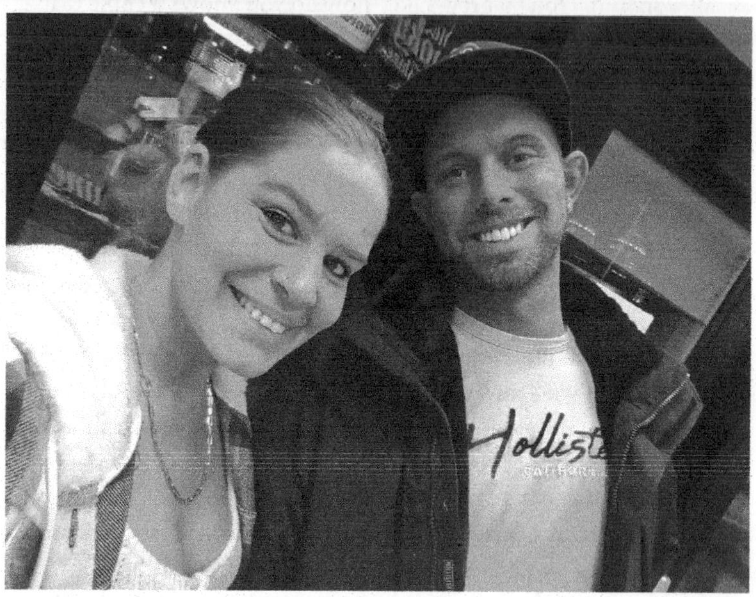

by Hailey Shields

Rain is the name of the daughter we lost in January of 2020. I do not know the reason for her passing away. I was three and a half months pregnant when I started bleeding at work. I left and immediately went to the emergency room. They did an ultrasound and bloodwork when I got there. I remember being worried that something was wrong with my baby. When I was getting the ultrasound, I kept waiting to hear a heartbeat but there was no sound. The woman who was doing it would not tell me anything. When I asked her why I could not hear a heartbeat she simply said, "The volume is turned down." I remember thinking that the baby I saw on the screen looked a lot smaller than it should have been. It took three hours of waiting before they told me that my baby had passed away five weeks prior.

At that time, the bleeding was light and I wasn't in any pain so they discharged me and sent me home. The next morning, I went to my OB and that's when three options were given to me. They gave me the option to wait for labor to happen naturally but they couldn't give me a time frame, and I had to work. I could have had a D&C two weeks later, but I didn't want her inside of me that long. I remember telling my husband, "I want her out. I want her out now." I also didn't want to risk the chance of going septic while waiting on the first two options. So, that left me with my last option, which was to do it at home with medicine: the abortion pill. I picked up the prescription, and on the 17th of January, I delivered her in my bathroom at home. I guess I was waiting for any sign of hope, or a way to change her fate, but I knew she was gone.

My husband and I took our girls to their grandma's house. We came home and I procrastinated taking the pill for hours after we picked it up from the pharmacy. When I did take it, it was so final. Although she was dead, I felt like I was finalizing her departure. It was terrible to know that I was taking the abortion pill for a baby we wanted.

This experience was disturbing, brutal, graphic, and terrifyingly painful in every way. I remember it every time I go into my bathroom. I was promised I wouldn't see her body when I delivered her, but I did see her. I saw ALL of her. I don't want to go into graphic details ... but I will, because these are the things I do not have the strength to say out loud.

I took the medicine and started crying. I started cramping and then the bleeding started. The cramps got worse. I realized then that I was having contractions. The bleeding got very heavy and I passed three blood clots the size of softballs. At one point, I was standing in my bathtub and the blood was pouring out of me; it sounded like running water when it hit my bathtub. I was scared and concerned. I called the on-call doctor and was told, "You're going to bleed like that for a couple of days." Against my better judgement, based on her advice, I stayed home instead of going to the emergency room.

I remember rolling around on the floor and in my bed and screaming because it hurt so badly. Even now, I still see red. My husband and I were slipping on the floor from all of the blood; it was everywhere. There were bloody handprints from holding onto the door and they were all over the sink. I remember my husband with towels trying to clean it all up as it was happening. It got to the point where he was on his hands and knees, drenched in sweat, with blood all over him and his clothes. He looked completely defeated. This lasted for four hours, and then everything got even more intense all at once.

I was sitting on the toilet when my water broke. I felt her come out and heard her hit the water. I looked down and started screaming, "It's the baby! It's my baby!" I was bawling my eyes out; I couldn't breathe. My heart hurt. Once I got her out of the toilet, I rinsed her off in the sink and just collapsed on the floor while I was holding her. When I did that, my husband lost it emotionally. I asked if he wanted to hold her and he just whispered, "I can't." I put her back in the toilet and flushed her.

I wish that I had held her longer. Had I been in a hospital setting, I know that the nurses would have given me options for her remains. I immediately regretted what I had done and it still bothers me to this day. I feel like I would have gotten closure if I had saved her body and buried her somewhere.

It was the most excruciating pain I have ever endured in my life. I look back and remember when it was all finally over. I just lay in my bed, naked, on a cold January night, with my window open. I felt the freezing air on my back. I was lightheaded and could barely move; then, I fell asleep.

When my first period came after my miscarriage, I was a wreck. Seeing the blood caught me off guard and triggered a lot of emotions. I'll never forget her or what she looked like when I held her. She was so peaceful and sweet. She fit perfectly in the palm of my hand. I was surprised by how small she was when I did see her because physically and mentally, I had carried her for three and a half months.

Is it possible to have PTSD over this? Every time I go into my bathroom, I see an image from that night. I would have been due July 24, 2020. Here I sit, daily anticipating ... what? I'm not crazy. On that day, nothing will happen, so why am I anticipating her due date so much? She's gone now. I'm hopeful things will get easier after that day. I've already requested to get off work on July 24th because I don't know how I'm going to feel.

I anticipated, waited for Rain's due date until it came. It was hard. I cried. I imagined holding her as a full-term baby and the day of happiness her arrival would have brought to us all. I was angry and I was sad. At the end of the day though, I did feel some relief from being able to let that obsession go. It wasn't until then that I truly started healing.

I did get a therapist and was diagnosed with PTSD. I have been seeing my therapist for over three months and all I have been able to tell her is that I lost a baby at home and that I have flashbacks from the night that it happened. I still can't really talk about it to anyone. I'm not sure how upset it will make me and I guess I am still not ready. I haven't grieved properly, and I am not sure that I will ever get closure. I don't think I will ever be the same. My thought on therapy for a long time was, if my own family, a group of people who love me can't comfort me, how can a complete stranger help? But I am grateful for my therapist. The validation and diagnosis of my PTSD was worth it.

Have you ever had a recurring dream? That is what my flashbacks are like. Rain is just a dream that will never come true. July 24, 2021, would have been her first birthday and I can't help but think about all of the milestones we will never get to experience with her. I will never hear her laugh or cry. I will never see her smile or get to know her. That is heartbreaking, and even after all of this time, I still think about her every day. I remember it like it happened yesterday.

Sometimes, losing a child can be hard on the relationship you have with your significant other. Everyone handles grief differently. My advice is just to be supportive in whatever way works for your spouse. My husband is an amazing father to our two daughters and an amazing husband. He hasn't talked about Rain. I'm still not sure he has fully grieved losing her either. He will always listen to me on my rough days and he tries to give me comfort. He never gets angry or annoyed when I talk about her. The only thing he has really said about what happened is that watching everything that I went through that night was scary. He said that it was hard for him to see all of the blood and watch me suffer. As difficult as it was for us to experience what we did, I am grateful that he was there for me that night and continues to be here for me.

Since losing Rain, we purchased a home and moved out of the apartment that held all of our bad memories. I got a tattoo of two red lilies with my living daughters' names above each one and I have an un-bloomed bud between them with Rain's name underneath it. I just completed my one-year of nursing prerequisites and I maintained the Dean's list for the entire year. In September, the application process for the nursing program will open up. I am hoping to be accepted so that I can accomplish my goal of becoming a registered nurse. And I am so grateful for the opportunity to share my story with all of you in this book.

If I were to give any advice to others who have gone through what I have, I would say: write a letter to your baby, seek help (because depression is a serious illness that can consume you completely). Talk about your baby as much as you want to, find local support groups or join groups on social media for parents who have lost children and say your baby's name out loud. Although you will never forget, it does get easier as time goes on. Some days will be harder than others, but try to embrace your feelings and your memories, because they are real, and they are all that we have left of our angels. Lastly, and most importantly, always remember that you are not alone.

Public Figures Share Their Personal Experiences To Help Others

Michelle Obama – *Miscarriage. Unknown/Undisclosed.*

> "I felt like I failed, because I didn't know how common miscarriages were, because we don't talk about them. We sit in our own pain, thinking that somehow we're broken. I think it's the worst thing that we do to each other as women, not share the truth about our bodies and how they work, and how they don't work."
>
> https://www.cbsnews.com/news/michelle-obama-reveals-miscarriage-daughters-malia-and-sasha-conceived-through-ivf/

19

My ANGEL IN HEAVEN

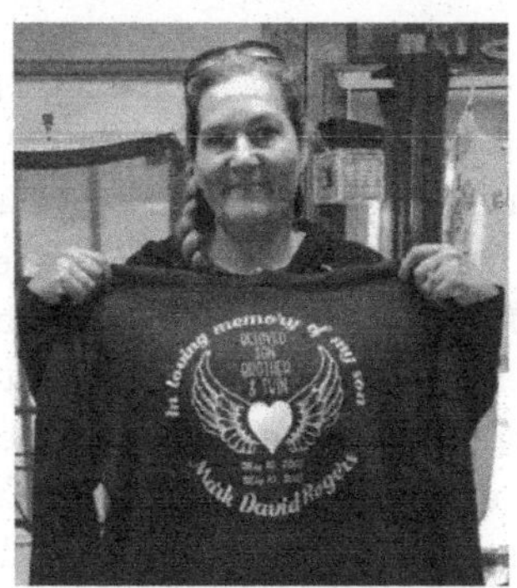
In loving memory of my son
BELOVED SON BROTHER & TWIN
Mark David Rogers

by Tammy Nichols-Rogers

I lost my son. I was pregnant with twins. I lost my son during the pregnancy, then his twin sister was born almost three months early. They had to fly her to Syracuse where she only had a 50/50 chance of making it. I prayed every day for her to please make it. After two and a half months of infections and blood transfusions, she was able to come home to me. But not a day goes by that I don't think of my son. I wonder if they would have been like each other. They weren't identical, but every day I just wonder, *Would he be just like her or would he be like my other boys?*

She came early due to their cords being tangled. I had to hold her in for an hour and a half until the Syracuse helicopter got there. After she was born, I got to hold her quickly and then I had to let her go. Then I was faced with having her brother removed. But God was with me that day because my son came out by himself so I didn't have to be cut open.

While they were growing in my belly, I got to feel both of them move around; it felt like butterflies. Even though he died at fifteen-and-a-half weeks, I still carried him until she arrived, almost three months early. She's 17 years old now and I still wonder every day about him. Every year on their birthday, we let balloons go. We write on the balloons and let him go.

Public Figures Share Their Personal Experiences To Help Others

Hilaria Baldwin – *16 weeks. Unknown/Undisclosed.*

"...While I am so blessed to have my babies, I have a few angels too. I had two miscarriages in a row in 2019–the second at 4 months. I was told 'it's just bad luck'...there is so much mystery why certain souls come into our lives and others do not. Today this baby I cried for [...] would have been about a year. April 23 was her 39 weeks. I had to go home and sleep with her inside of me for one more night before having surgery the next. This was the last photo of my girls at the time. My face so swollen—I remember being surprised that the body could make so many tears—kept on thinking I'd run out of them. [...]I took [a photo] a day or so before I found out I had lost her. I looked tired, but happy...celebrating the pregnancy.

A year since she was due, my Edu and Lucia are constant companions, but I think of the babies I lost daily. Resigned and respectful of how my life has unfolded. Allowing for gratitude and grief, wholeness and longing to be the dualities of my reality.

We all have different fertility/infertility stories and there are so many ways we can become parents. Being a parent truly is caring in the deepest way for another soul...through that giving energy we nurture ourselves and fill the world with love. I am just as much a mother to my Angel babies as I am to the ones I can physically hold in my arms. If you are struggling or have struggled—or will struggle, know that you are not alone...if it serves you, connect with others as you grieve. We are a mighty bunch who carry this heaviness in our hearts—and together we can lighten each other's load through support and understanding."

Instagram https://www.instagram.com/p/COBWEJjMctT/?utm_source=ig_embed&ig_rid=f8ffd437-68ed-45d0-a496-5a94228a873f

20

Whispers of Comfort

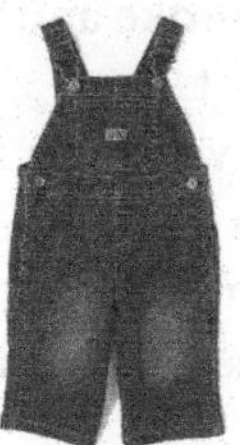

by Dee-Anna Janku

I lost my first baby at 17 weeks into my pregnancy. The events of those days are etched in my mind and seem like a mix of a nightmare and reality.

My husband, Scott, and I had only been married for a few months when we learned we were pregnant. We were looking forward to having a baby, our parents' first grandchild. Scott was taking college courses and I was working a temporary job. The minute they found out I was pregnant, I lost that job.

As I interviewed for another job, I kept my pregnancy a secret. I was hired by a man named Larry to be a secretary at his HVAC shop. Shortly after starting the job, on one of my days off, I had an appointment with my OBGYN. He sent me over for an ultrasound the next day. I was excited to learn the gender of our baby and disappointed that my husband couldn't make it to the appointment.

The ultrasound tech called in the doctor. Her words were abrupt and lacked all the tenderness one would hope for. "Your baby is a boy and just like we thought, he no longer has a heartbeat. You have two choices. We can either do an abortion or wait for the child to pass naturally." Everything in me recoiled at the word "abortion." I stuttered out that I would wait and I left the office, alone. That was in 2001 and I didn't yet carry a cell phone with me. I went home, alone, and cried and waited for my husband to get home. I told him and no one else. We waited. Two days later, while at church, I began cramping and bleeding. My husband took me to the ER.

They hooked me up to morphine as a painkiller before taking me into surgery for a D&C. This is where my memory gets fuzzy. My husband tells me I had a strong reaction, ripping out my IV and cursing at the nurses. I never swear, so he knew it was the drugs. I remember nothing until I woke up the next morning at home. My sister was there. She told me that she had helped my husband get me home. I literally had no memory of that.

The state we were living in required an autopsy to determine the cause of death since the baby, whom we named Malachai, had passed after 16 weeks. They discovered that Malachai had cancer and decided they needed to do a second D&C to ensure that no cancerous tissue was left behind. I again have no memory until waking up at home, with my sister there just like before. We were broke and Scott needed to work. He wanted to be with me, but he couldn't.

The first night at home, I woke up from a nightmare, drenched in sweat. My husband said that, in my sleep, I had accused them of "stealing my baby." My dreams gave me away. It was the first nightmare on the first night of more than five months of nightmares that would come, relentlessly reminding me.

I tried to go back to work the next day, but Larry fired me for "lying" to him by not telling him I was pregnant. I needed to mourn but didn't think I had permission. It seemed like most of the world didn't count this as a real loss, just because he was never born. Most close family members never acknowledged that it happened. Others made thoughtless comments about how it was "better" that it had happened now, before we knew him and, "It would have been harder if you had lost him later." It was hard in the moment. It was hard regardless of the fact that we'd never met him. He existed. He was our child. We lost him. We didn't expect this. No one does.

There was no service, no sympathy, no fanfare. All we had was a shoebox of items we'd purchased for him, items we still have; a cute overall outfit that all of our children have worn, and couple of other tiny mementos.

As word got out to our church family, my phone started ringing. First it was an older woman who shared that she too had lost a baby at just 8 weeks and never got over it. "Back in my time," she told me, "No one mentioned it. But I wanted you to know that you aren't alone." Then, another woman, whose children are grown, shared her story; then, a friend that was also newlywed. Before the week was up, I'd heard from at least a dozen women. Each one shared and found comfort in sharing as much as they provided comfort to me.

Those days are fuzzy, but I remember the stories of those women. I can still hear their whispers, as if they were sharing a secret with me. So many had never talked about it. They were guarded and yet open, with an understanding that only one who had gone through it could truly possess. They encouraged me to mourn. They assured me that my thoughts were normal. They told me again and again that I wasn't alone.

I also remember talking to a group of women once and, needing to be comforted, I told them that I had lost a baby at seventeen weeks. I knew they thought I meant that he was born and had come home with us before we lost him. I let them think it. It was easier. They understood the pain that I must have been feeling and mourned with me differently from anyone else. I mourned differently than I had before, and with that mourning came healing.

My nightmares only stopped as we packed our bags and moved across the country. We were halfway between here and there, in a grocery store restroom, when I took a test revealing I was pregnant again. To be honest, I spent that entire pregnancy waiting for it to end, wondering which day we would get the news that she no longer had a heartbeat. It wasn't until I held her in my arms that I finally agreed it was going to be okay.... At least for this baby. But none of our children would "replace" Malachai. We now have five children with us and three more waiting with Malachai in heaven. I still think of Malachai often and do the math. He'd be 19 years old now and probably in college like his little sister.

I have learned, through many hard days with children who have multiple medical issues, that as parents, we have one job: to prepare our children for the day they will meet Jesus. It's the one thing that is certain: all of our children are dying. I am dying. So is my husband. But one day, we will all stand before our Creator and the only thing that will matter is if he knows us. This is our promised future.

I have learned that death is expected; it happens to the best of us, and it isn't fitting, as Christians, that when we face death (our own or that of a loved one) that we become like Chicken Little, running about crying that, "The sky is falling!" Death in this world is expected, but true hope is found in an eternity in God's presence. This greater hope grounds me in my darkest days. God had a plan for our good; not in spite of the hard, but in the hard. He doesn't take the hard and turn it around to become good. He intended the hard for our good and His glory. This truth gives me incredible hope regardless of what each day might bring.

PUBLIC FIGURES SHARE THEIR PERSONAL EXPERIENCES TO HELP OTHERS

BROOKE SHIELDS – *Miscarriage. Cervical dysplasia.*

"We were crushed. Up till then, I thought simply because it was time and I wanted to have a baby, it would work.

"Maybe I'll never know why it happened. But it made me understand the difference between wanting to have a baby and truly wanting to be a mother."

In a 2003 interview with People https://www.insider.com/celebrities-who-had-miscarriages-2018-11#brooke-shields-experienced-a-pregnancy-loss-after-undergoing-ivf-treatment-22

21

Alexander Rodriguez

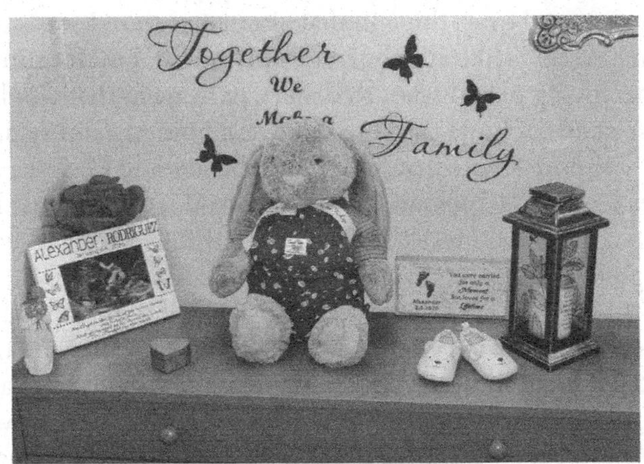

by Silvia Rodriguez

I experienced my loss on February 4, 2020. At my seventeen-and-a-half-week appointment, I heard those awful words: "I'm sorry. There's no heartbeat." My son had passed away sometime around fifteen and a half weeks. I chose to deliver him and was able to do so at eighteen weeks. It was then discovered that his umbilical cord was wrapped around his neck four times.

It's been a rough road. Today I feel okay but most of the time, I wake up wishing I hadn't.

I hate the word miscarriage ... I didn't miscarry him. That word makes me feel worse. I was supposed to be his safest place and instead I was his death; I was his tomb. I couldn't save him. I couldn't protect him. Miscarry!? Did I not do everything in my power? Yes, I did. I started drinking more water, taking vitamins, walking more, trying to lower my blood pressure naturally. How is that miscarrying? It's a medical term, I know, but I HATE it. My son had an accident, one where I couldn't help him; however, I can't help but feel guilty. I can't stop wondering if I drank something that made him hyper enough to entangle himself. Perhaps I was sleeping too much on my back. Perhaps it was the cold drink I had. I will never know.

I hate that society was quick to tell me I was carrying my child but as soon as he died, my child became an "At least this and that," or, "It wasn't even a baby," etc. I hate all the attempts to comfort because in reality, they hurt more. "At least" – There's no, "At least." There's no lesson to be learned. There's no silver lining to losing Alexander. God's plan? What a cruel way of telling me he loves me, giving me a child only for me to lose him and watch inept mothers neglecting, abandoning, abusing, or even murdering their own. Yet here I am, empty arms and shattered heart, missing my son and everything in that alternate future I was supposed to have. To me, it seems like an arbitrary punishment. I'm not sure how that could be his loving plan. I want to believe in heaven; that would give me even a false sense of hope that I will see and hold my son again and this nightmare will end. (Note that I respect all beliefs and I believe that whatever makes a person happy and a better person is great. I just had many doubts and considered myself agnostic until this. Now I just can't believe even though I *want* to.)

I hate that people can't show sympathy even if they don't fully understand. I mean, before I experienced it, I couldn't fully imagine the impact it truly had but I still showed sympathy and said an almost rehearsed, "I'm so sorry for your loss." In reality, there's not much to say anyway. But to receive, "You still cry?" I wanted to scream all the negative thoughts in my head but I knew I didn't mean it. I was just angry that she, being a mom and expecting, couldn't at least begin to understand that I didn't lose a pair of shoes. I lost my son, MY SON! For goodness sake, even my best male friend, who is not a father, cried with me and for Alexander.

I hate that society undermines these losses; that we grieve in silence because it's frowned upon to mourn or grieve over something we didn't have. Well, I did have a child growing inside. Just because the outside world didn't meet him does not mean Alexander didn't exist. He did exist and was NOT a figment of my imagination.

I have a nineteen-year old and I keep going for him, but losing Alexander has been the most painful event I've ever had to endure. I have experienced other heartbreaks, depression, and losses. None were remotely like this loss and agony. I thought I knew pain until I lost him. I feel it has broken me in a whole new way that I didn't know existed. A million words can't describe this immense pain and helplessness. No one is ever prepared to say goodbye to a child regardless of their age (gestational or otherwise).

I hate all this pain. It's exhausting to cry, to hurt, to live with the life that was lost. Lost in life, lost in thoughts, lost in grief. I am no longer me. I've lost so much more than a pregnancy.

I will someday have to accept it as an unfortunate event that has changed my life, my thinking, my emotions. For now, I hurt, I cry, I mourn the loss and the could/would have beens. This pandemic also doesn't help. I can't grieve or mourn but then again, I suppose it comes and goes. One moment I'm fine and the next I'm crying my heart out.

I am a 40-year-old woman. Learning that I had become pregnant was scary yet exciting, like when I was pregnant with my now nineteen-year-old, Martin. I began to plan, and purchase items including clothes and diapers. Martin didn't care what gender we got; he just wanted a sibling. I had raised my now-seven-year-old nephew, Roberto, and I was nervous to tell him because he is like my child. He practically lived with me until the age of six when my brother moved to a different state. Roberto was a bit reluctant, or rather shocked, but hours later, he demonstrated his embracement of being a "big Brother." I video chatted with him and gave him updates, shared ultrasound pictures and videos. Roberto was so excited that he would have a "sibling" to teach and play with. He, too, had plans, just as Martin had his own, I had mine, and so did everyone around me.

I shared the news with my immediate family on Christmas Eve. Shocked and in disbelief and happy-crying, they jumped for joy and hugged me while looking in awe at ultrasound pictures and videos. My aunt and cousins also began buying items and making plans. Everyone was over the moon, with smiling hearts.

I can still feel the joy I felt when I first saw Alexander's tiny body and form that looked like a blob and heard his heartbeat. That *lub-dub* sound made it all real. I would be a mother of two. I began to cry with love and happiness. I heard life within me. Soon after, we used Blueberry as a nickname while still not knowing the gender. Blueberry would become Xotchil if a girl and Alexander if a boy. Several appointments, including the genetic and NTS (Nuchal Translucency Scan), came and went. All was normal and perfect. My baby was going to be a boy. Now our plans included more gender-based choices, although, I must admit, those choices were mostly on clothes since we would still have done activities such as fishing and hiking had he been a girl.

Next up was my anatomy scan. Right before that, I had a routine check up. My OB asked the routine questions and asked if I was now feeling movement. I was, indeed, although, over the last few days, I had felt less. I spoke to my mom about it but comforted myself with the thought that maybe it was because he was still so small. My OB asked if I wanted a vaginal or an abdominal ultrasound. I confessed that it didn't matter. She proceeded to place gel on the wand and glide it across my lower abdomen. Immediately, I knew something was wrong. I could not find the flicker. I must have been in shock, perhaps in denial, because it didn't hit me like a ton of rocks. Tears began to gather but I was hopeful that the ultrasound wand would get better placement and we would see it. My OB was still quiet, searching for signs of life. She tapped on one side and that is when I knew. A tear rolled off my cheek as she said, "I'm so sorry. There's no heartbeat." (If you ask me, that phrase should be banned from all languages.)

While my doctor gave me some time to process, I texted my best friend in order to then review my options. "I don't like this f-ing joke," She replied. I shot back, "It's not a joke; my baby is dead and has been dead for two weeks now." I called my son and my mom. Both could not comprehend what I was telling them. I walked to my car, that indescribable walk of shame, guilt, loneliness, wonder, emptiness. During that awfully long, three-minute walk, it was all sinking in. Desperation began to set in. I felt defeated, trapped in a room without windows, without doors. All was dark and cloudy. The thunder in my head was loud but I could still hear my heart breaking. That day was January 29, 2020.

After reviewing my options, and having a confirmatory scan on January 30, 2020, I could not fathom the idea of my son in pieces and not being able to see or hold him. I chose to deliver him. That option gave me the opportunity to hold, kiss, sing, and love my son. I got to have him with me for a few precious hours until the funeral home picked him up.

During the month that followed, I lived in limbo, a world that is neither here nor there. I was wanting to give up and die but needing to stay for Martin and for Roberto. I was torn because they deserved a happy mom/godmother.

My son, my mom, my cousin, and three friends have helped me cope. I am extremely grateful that they have been so patient and understanding. They check up on me and let me vent, self-loathe, even self-pity, and simply grieve. They have provided the true meaning of unconditional love and support, from making dinner for me to simply asking how I am doing; then reminding me that I am loved and needed by them all and advising me to take my time, day by day, or moment by moment if need be.

I have this great need to "prove" that my son was real. I have contemplated starting a non-profit to gather more resources for others. I just don't know how to start. For now, I have gotten a tattoo (and I plan on getting more) in his honor. I have started crocheting and making tiny blankets to put at least ten care boxes together for other loss moms. I plan to donate them to the hospital where my son was birthed. Joining loss groups has also helped because even though I have a great support system and no matter how much they say they understand, it all feels so lonely. I have also reached out for help and I am taking antidepressants. I still cry often but can only imagine: *If I hadn't started them, would I even be here?* Another thing I have done to help me cope is to sign up for bereavement doula classes. It has been months since I signed up but I cry when I start reading the material. I'm glad both classes are self-paced. One day, I will have the ability to provide some support to another grieving mother and her family. On his one-year anniversary (and every year thereafter), I plan to anonymously buy birthday cakes for a child of Alexander's age.

Things need to change. I hope to muster the courage to begin opening up publicly to spread awareness.. We suffer so much and the least we deserve is the compassion and space to grieve instead of being shut down, ignored, or dismissed as if we are overly dramatic in making this a big deal. This IS a big deal. Like I said, I did not lose a pair of shoes or keys, I LOST MY SON. WE have all lost our children.

22

Declan and Devlan

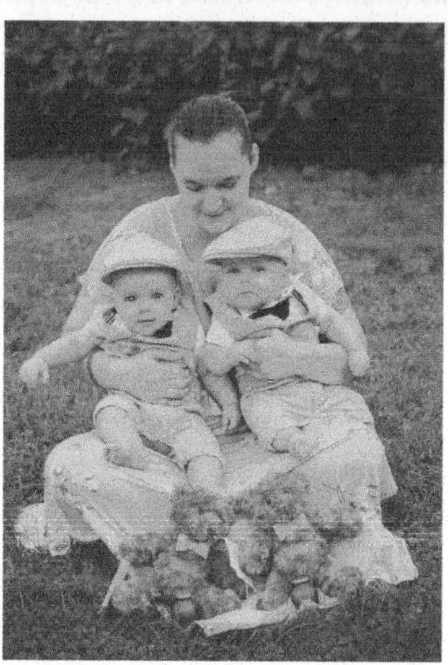

by Marsha Sparks

I want to share my story so no one else has to experience this type of unnecessary pain. I want to start by explaining that I was pregnant with twin boys and that they were diagnosed with TTTS (Twin-to-Twin Transfusion Syndrome), meaning they had one placenta and abnormal blood vessels.

I had seen a specialist in Cincinnati, Ohio, a two-and-a-half-hour drive from my home, but at the time they felt surgery was too risky for the babies and decided to continue to monitor the situation. On November 23, 2019, I began to leak amniotic fluid, so I went to the closest E.R. (Baptist Health in Richmond, KY) to be sure. That is where I saw Dr. Cody G.

The point of going to the E.R. close to home was to check the fluid and see if I needed to return to Cincinnati to the specialist for surgery. I explained my babies' condition and that I was being monitored in Cincinnati. Dr. G. refused to do the test on the fluid; instead, he did an ultrasound where he did see the fluid was actually low. He still refused to check the fluid levels to know if my babies were losing fluid and how much. He said the fluid of Baby B was low, but that it didn't matter if it was amniotic fluid because I was only seventeen weeks pregnant. He determined their heartbeats were fine and they both had fluid so I could go home, since I probably wasn't leaking.

On Tuesday, November 26, I had an appointment with my high-risk doctor, at Baptist Health in Lexington. I still felt like I was losing fluid so I expressed my concerns. He conducted an ultrasound and measured the fluid. It showed Baby A had gone from 8 cm of fluid to 4.1. Dr. M. said it was probably just correcting itself and I probably was not losing fluid. However, I told him I had been gushing fluid. He said everything was great because they had a heartbeat and then he sent me home, still not testing the fluid. As a first-time pregnant woman, I was at a loss as to how to proceed, so I took their advice and went home and tried not to worry.

The following morning, November 27 at one A.M., I started having contractions that came every five minutes, so, after two A.M., my family took me to the nearest E.R. that delivered babies, Baptist Health in Richmond. The nurse put me in a room and I explained what was going on. She recognized me and asked, "Weren't you just here this past Saturday?" I said, "Yes," and she said she would let the doctor know what was going on. To my disappointment and surprise, the E.R. doctor was, once again, Dr. G!

Forty-five minutes later, he came in and asked what was going on. I explained the fluid leaking, contractions, and pressure. He said, "Okay," and walked out the door, with no exams. The nurse came in with an IV and I asked if Dr. G was going to check on my babies or call an OB. She said, "No, he just wants to start an IV and get an ultrasound." There wasn't an ultrasound tech there so we had to wait for one to arrive. I told her I needed to use the restroom before she started the IV. I went to the restroom but I couldn't use the toilet because I could literally see my baby's head; he was ready to come out!

I told the nurse what was happening and she told the doctor. I heard him mumble something and then he laughed. He walked in at approximately 3:30 A.M. and said, "Well, I thought you had to go pee." I explained what I had told the nurse and his response was, "Well, if you need to push, you can do so in the bathroom because they are going to be dead anyway!"

At this point I was begging him to just check me and call the OB. I told him I was worried about my own safety since I have epilepsy, Ehlers-Danlos Syndrome, and POTS. He responded that he was not calling the OB because at 3:30 A.M., labor is NOT an emergency, and if I needed it, he could bring in a bedside toilet instead. I asked once more for the OB. He again refused and said it didn't matter; and that if I did not like it, I was free to leave because it wasn't a jail.

Finally, at 4 A.M., the ultrasound tech arrived, performed a scan, and determined that one of the babies was in my cervix and a heartbeat could not be found for either. By this time the pressure was so bad, I requested a bedside toilet. The nurse brought it in and while I was sitting on it, Dr. G. came in and said, "Well, I'm sorry. I guess I should have listened because you were right, but I'm having a bad night." He walked out and my first baby was born in a bedside toilet with no doctor in the room.

The nurse asked me if I wanted to get back in the bed and I explained I couldn't because I could feel my baby still attached to the cord. The nurse left and told Dr. G. He sent her back to ask if I wanted to pull it the rest of the way out or if I want him to do it. He came in and tried to pull and realized that wasn't going to work, since I had another baby in waiting. At this point, I had been sitting on a toilet, still in labor, for 30 minutes. Dr. G. then, *finally*, called the OB because he didn't know what to do.

Labor and delivery (L&D) nurses arrived at my room around 5 A.M.; they helped get me back in bed and deliver baby B at 5:10 A.M. However, the OB was not there because he hadn't had time to arrive yet.

Dr. G. couldn't get the placenta delivered so the L&D nurses told him they were taking me upstairs. At that point, I started hemorrhaging while waiting for the OB to arrive. The nurses were getting very nervous and, at one time, actually called to check his location. My blood pressure dropped down to 66 over 40 and a lot of trauma happened. I reported Dr. G. to the hospital that same day. But so far, nothing has been done.

I want everyone to understand that I underwent fertility treatments to get pregnant. My twins were Declan (7 oz.) and Devlan (6.4 oz.) and they were both loved. They were born prematurely at 18 weeks+1 day.

Since the loss of my twins, I have tried two more rounds of fertility treatments but both have been unsuccessful. My main coping mechanisms have been crocheting items for other loss parents to have at the hospital for their babies, loving on my nephews, and I have not given up on getting pregnant or getting justice for my twins.

Public Figures Share Their Personal Experiences To Help Others

Beyonce – *Multiple miscarriages. Unknown/Undisclosed.*

> "About two years ago, I was pregnant for the first time. And I heard the heartbeat, which was the most beautiful music I ever heard in my life.
>
> "I picked out names. I envisioned what my child would look like . . . I was feeling very maternal.
>
> "I flew back to New York to get my check up -- and no heartbeat. Literally the week before I went to the doctor, everything was fine, but there was no heartbeat.
>
> "I went into the studio and wrote the saddest song I've ever written in my life. And it was actually the first song I wrote for my album. And it was the best form of therapy for me, because it was the saddest thing I've ever been through."
>
> https://www.today.com/parents/beyonce-opens-miscarriage-saddest-thing-ive-ever-been-through-1b8198402

23

A LETTER TO MY ANGELS

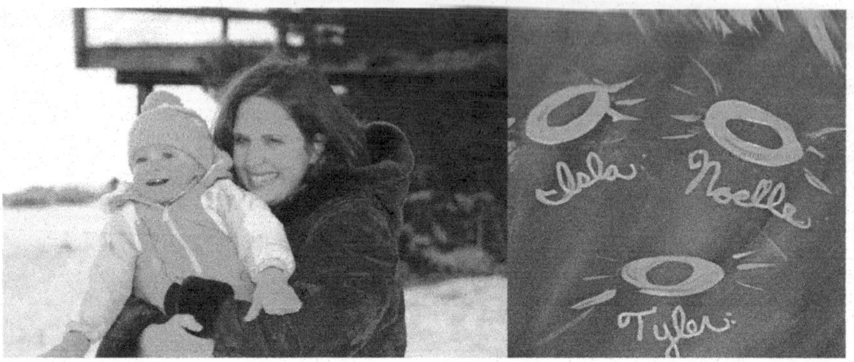

by Justina Engen

I have written a letter to all of my living children about their births. These letters are wonderful little pieces of my heart, weaved together into stories that climax with incredibly wonderful and happy events and outcomes that I will treasure forever. I have shared these stories with my living children and really, anyone who would listen. These stories are celebrated and cherished and have helped me create a community around my journey of motherhood.

However, I also have other stories to tell ... other stories that have touched me so deeply, that changed me just as much, if not exponentially more, than my two living childrens' testimonies. These are stories of loss, of trauma, of tragedy, and of deep loneliness. But these stories are also of love, desire, and deep, deep sacrifice in bringing forth the true miracle of life.

I've sat down multiple times to write the story of losing my angels: a baby girl, born unexpectedly midway through my second pregnancy; another baby (whom I believe in my heart was a girl), whose heart stopped beating at 12 weeks' gestation; and my only son, who traumatically entered this world at 14 weeks only to leave his placenta behind and cause me lots of health issues that I still have to this day. Seven years later, I am still fighting to regain the woman I once was.

While I will never get to share these stories with them, I've wanted to write these stories to honor them and to heal myself. It really wasn't until I acknowledged my oldest angel's life, her birth and her death, and the life and death of her younger little sister, that I was able to move forward with my life. And then, my son's birth and death brought a whole new wave of emotions and challenges that caused me to feel, even while being tragically over-experienced in this field, completely overwhelmed and blind-sided by his story, which led to a deep depression that made it hard to even focus on the skills I had learned with my previous girls.

I knew I needed to tell their stories; however, every time I sat down to write, I hit major walls. At first, it was the pain of reliving these tragic and horrific experiences that, initially, I didn't even count as births. Why would anyone want to read about this? This was my burden to bear and no one else would understand.

Then, as time went on, I became more and more interested in writing this piece, but the words never seemed right. At first, they were angry, focusing on all the injustices I endured and the journey of losing my faith in many things, including my body and my spiritual beliefs. But all these words were focusing on my pain and anger, rather than honoring my babies. I wanted to honor them and find a way to be proud of their short time in my life; and how they have truly changed it forever.

After I wrote my rainbow baby's incredibly positive birth story, with highlights of my angels' lives, I really wanted to write this story in a way that would explain how my life was touched and how much these little humans have changed me into a deeper, stronger, more compassionate woman. But how could I put that into words? I couldn't tell their stories like my others, because my memories of these births are shattered pieces of my heart that I have slowly been picking up and weaving back into my life in such a way that I can live with them and move forward.

I wrote the stories of my first two angels two years after their births, after I had experienced the incredible healing birth of my now-ten-year-old, rainbow child. That was before my son was born. At that time, I honestly felt like I had overcome that tragic season of my life. I was able to talk and share about my two girls as if they had lived and were watching over our family, protecting us.

Then my pregnancy with my son came, and tragically ended, and left me, and my very tired body, in a sea of despair. So much so that I stopped writing altogether. I had lost my way and it was all I could do to keep my marriage, my young, living childrens' basic needs met, and myself alive. I couldn't process this trauma, so I turned my back on the community that had supported me through my previous losses and the birth of my living babies and it's not until now, over seven years later, that I am opening this chapter again to honor him and his sisters in the way that they were meant to be honored.

Baby Girl 1: We now have named her Isla

"I'm sorry, it looks like you are going to lose this pregnancy." The OBGYN stated very matter-of-factly to me, with no hint of emotion in her voice. I really couldn't believe the words coming from this woman's mouth, whom I had met less than 5 minutes before and had supposedly been monitoring my progress for the preceding 12 twelve hours.

"WHAT? I just felt the baby moving," I said in utter disbelief, holding back tears. As they rushed to get an ultrasound, I recounted all the recent events. *Had I missed something? Had they missed something? Why was I losing this baby?* No one told me this was even a possibility.... I was alone, away from my twenty-month-old daughter for the first time in her life, with my feet in the air, waiting for what I had thought was going to be a simple surgery, while my husband was sitting in an airport over a thousand miles away.

I had just had a prenatal visit less than a week before. I also called the midwife-on-call for a simple, weird mucous with a streak of blood in it. At first, I was told to "ignore it" and not to leave my twenty-month-old on a stormy Friday night to wait in an ER for hours for "probably nothing." I still debated after the midwife called back, telling me that we would probably all feel better if I went and had an ultrasound "just in case."

Even after sitting in the ER for hours, watching all the auto-accident victims and homeless people looking for a dry place to stay for the night being seen ahead of me, and finally getting an ultrasound slightly after midnight, I didn't worry. I remember joking with the ultrasound tech after hearing the heartbeat and hearing the words the ER doctor said: "Your bag is bulging, but the baby is fine."

I remember calling my husband and telling him that, "worst case scenario," I was going to have to have surgery and need bedrest. I told him to go to bed so I could see him the next day when he flew home. Even after being admitted, and placed on my head in hopes of my bag receding, I worried more about my twenty-month-old, recently weaned baby at home, who had never gone to bed for the night without me. And there was the ominous question the nurses constantly asked me, "Is there fetal movement?" *Okay, I must be fine.... My baby is moving ... how could this pregnancy be ending?*

The ultrasound confirmed the doctor's prognosis: the baby was so low in the pelvis that they couldn't even detect the sac. And then she repeated, "I'm sorry, but you are going to lose this baby ... there is nothing we can do." The tears I had been barely holding back flooded my eyes. I somehow managed to call my mom, and uttered incoherently, "I'm going to lose the baby." I don't even remember what she said, but I knew she was on her way.

I then had to call Leif, my sweet husband, who had recently endured the tragedy of losing both his grandparents, and I know would have driven all night in sub-zero temperatures and fought with airlines to get home if he knew this was a possibility. A man, on his way home to be comforted by his pregnant wife and toddler, had to be told by his scared and devastated wife that he would never meet his second baby.

He answered the phone, expecting to comfort and encourage me, while trying to hide his worry about our previous call. When I told him the news through my sobs, silence fell on the other end of the phone. He told me later that he was surrounded by family, but suddenly wanted to be alone or at least moving towards me. He didn't want to talk; he just wanted to move ... but all he could do was wait for a plane. I hung up the phone, and my mom was there. With tears in her eyes, she gave me a hug and a kiss. I don't know if we exchanged words, but I was so glad and angry that she was there. I wanted her, but I wanted my husband more. *Why isn't he here?* The room was full of people: the OB, nurses, lab techs ... but I felt alone.

The OB talked to my mom, asked me some questions about my medical history and then popped off some reason why this was happening. "Incompetent Cervix" was the term constantly used and, boy, did I feel incompetent. *How could my body expel such a lively, active little being? Were those little wiggles and kicks I felt only hours before cries for help, rather than what I thought were measures of comfort?*

They told me that the best thing to do was, "Let nature take its course," and to page the nurse when "it" was over. They offered me pain meds, which I declined because I didn't have any physical pain and I didn't want the pain to go away; I wanted to feel every ounce of pain ... it wouldn't come close to the emotional pain I was in. One thing I did ask for was water, which they denied in case I needed surgery to remove the baby. They explained what a D&C was and then suddenly the room was empty.

My mom asked me a bunch of questions that I answered, "I don't know" to, and then I asked if she could see the amniotic sack. She could; my bag was literally bulging out ... I was delivering this baby. She asked me if I wanted a mirror and I told her, "Yes." I looked and there I saw my body expelling what looked like a little, dark-red balloon. I sat and cried ... not wanting to talk, just wanting to cry.

Every time the nurse came in, I could read the look on her face and the tone in her voice; she was truly apologetic and baffled that she hadn't seen any signs. She told me that with every check she did, she saw no reasons for concern, especially because I wasn't showing any signs of pain and I was feeling the baby move. She brought me warm blankets and left me to stare out the window at the stormy day that truly reflected how I felt inside.

The doctor came in again and told me about what would probably happen. She said that because the baby was younger than twenty weeks, there would be no attempts to revive the baby, and that while I was close to twenty weeks, this would be considered a miscarriage rather than a stillbirth. I was later told by others that I was "lucky" that it was earlier than twenty weeks, and I didn't have to name the baby, or sign a stillbirth and death certificate. As if somehow, magically, at twenty weeks, I would have loved that baby more, or that by those acts of grief it would have hurt more. Looking back, I wish I had been offered some of those options in a kind and gentle manner. Because, in that moment, somehow, I was afraid to love that baby for real, to honor her and myself as I should. So, I just sat there, in complete despair and shock, waiting for "it" to be over.

Shortly thereafter, I felt my body give a short, little push. I felt it again and slowly something slipped out onto my bed. I told my mom, who had no clue I had just given birth. She looked and then went and got the nurse. It was only for a moment, but I saw the caul that my baby was nestled so snugly inside. It was so surreal; everything just came out, smoothly and calmly. No heavy pushing, no emergency, no anything, except pure sadness. The nurse came in, wrapped the caul up, and took it away, seeming to assume I didn't want to see it. I wish I had stopped her. I wish she had offered me some words of encouragement to see my creation, but I did feel like it would be too painful; and I figured she was sparing me that pain.

I then cried hard. It was over. My sweet baby was born into the arms of angels on 12/12/09 at 12:12 p.m., less than two hours after the news that I was going to lose her, and less than a day from the first symptoms. I called Leif and only had one phrase, "It's over." We cried together, wishing we could hold each other, wishing we were both somewhere of comfort rather than me in a cold, dreary hospital room, surrounded by women giving birth to live, healthy babies and him, sitting in an airport, waiting to board a plane, only hours too late to see his baby girl.

The OB then came in and asked if I wanted to know the sex. I looked at my mom and then said, "Yes." It was a girl. The OB said she looked "normal," with no visible defects. The OB then asked if I wanted to see her. I then also said, "Yes." They brought her in on a tucks pad ... no blanket, no clothes, no anything. I looked at her and marveled in both pain and amazement. She was so much bigger than I had imagined her. At 18 weeks and 3 days, she looked bigger than the preemies they portray on television. She had fingernails. I'll never forget how her fingernails looked. She was a real baby; she looked so peaceful, but also so lifeless. It was like looking at a shell. She had been so lively inside me; I had felt her at 15 weeks and her dad had felt her move at 16 weeks. Now, she had no movement, no life... she was no longer there.

I also marveled at her umbilical cord, wrapped twice around her neck. They told me it wasn't the reason she passed, although others believed it was. I know now that it wasn't. The cord was absolutely amazing, a true lifeline to my baby girl, an iridescent clear with red and blue veins spinning along it. I will always remember that; it was the one thing at that moment that I was truly proud I had created.

The nurse then asked if I wanted to hold her. I hadn't thought of that and almost panicked. *Should I hold her? Would I feel more pain? She was no longer there, but would she feel more lifelike if I did hold her? Would I regret holding her, or not holding her? What did my mom think?* I burst into tears and cried, "I don't know!" The nurse immediately hugged me and told me it was okay, that I had never done this before and there was no way for me to know. I then picked my baby up. She was so light I could barely feel her. I held her close to me and cried. My mom held me and we both cried. Looking back, I wish I had spent more time holding her, taking her in, and letting my mom hold me, but it was all so lacking in life that I felt uncomfortable. My baby was gone, and I never got to meet her; she was the shell of a person that once almost was. I didn't know where she was, but she was no longer with me.

I called Leif again; he asked if they could wait for him to see her. I asked the nurses, but they couldn't really give me an answer. I don't think they could have discharged me without "taking care" of the body, or at least I got that feeling, so I asked if I could take pictures. My mom took pictures on her camera and then she laid my baby at the end of my bed.

I wish now that I would have held her until they took her from me, but I was so lost in a blur that I didn't know what to do. It was like I wanted permission to love my baby no matter her state. I felt like I had to guard myself from acknowledging her birth and her life, so I just lay there, and stared at her, and cried; and then I just stared, because there were no tears left.

A few hours later, the nurse brought in a plate of food and I told her I wasn't hungry, just thirsty. Suddenly, I realized I had eaten the whole plate and was asking for more water. Then, they got me up to make sure I could use the restroom and told me that I could go home shortly. My sister brought me a clean pair of clothes and I showered and then packed up, ready to leave. I was scared to see moms with babies or hear the joy of birth around me, but I didn't. All was quiet. The nurse hugged me with tears in her eyes and told me I did wonderfully. I didn't understand what she meant, but I do now: I had endured birth, life, death, and loss all in a matter of hours, which seemed like a matter of minutes; and I was still alive, walking out of the hospital.

I arrived home minutes before my dad left to pick Leif up from the airport. I took another shower and then my sister brushed my hair. My toddler climbed into my arms and fell asleep. It was pouring rain outside. I sat in the dark living room, holding my living baby, praying, worrying that my husband wouldn't walk through that door. I just couldn't bear to lose him too, but I was almost expecting it. My life was shattered, and I had no idea how to pick up the pieces, except to expect more devastation.

Leif did get home. I think we ate. We then went into the guest bedroom, looked at her pictures, and cried together. We cried for what felt like hours. We slept and then woke up and cried more. The days following seemed to be a blur. Everyone asked me how I felt. Physically, I felt fine, my body acted as though nothing had happened. No one outside of my close circle would have even suspected that days before, I was almost halfway through my pregnancy. I felt like I wanted to run a marathon and yell and scream and cry and sleep and collapse all at the same time. Words meant as encouragement enraged me. "At least you're okay," made me furious. I screamed at my mom, telling her I wanted to feel pain, I wanted to be physically hurt, because I felt like I was dying inside.

One of the midwives called and I talked with her for hours. She seemed to get it. She had been the one on call the night I started showing signs, who told me to "ignore it" and then called back fifteen minutes later, telling me to go get an ultrasound "just in case." She told me it was okay for me to want this experience to feel momentous, and that she wished she could do more. She gave me her personal phone number and email and told me to call for any reason. That in itself was the most comfort anyone, other than my husband and daughter, could give me, just to tell me that she was there for me. She didn't have to be, but she was there.

The midwives also told me that their office would be calling to set up an appointment with a peritonologist to look into reasons this could have happened. The maternal-fetal medicine specialist was also a true blessing; she didn't know me, or my husband, but she treated me like she had been through the pain with me. In the months that followed, she ordered all the tests in the world, but she was also the first person to admit that she simply didn't know why. She said that sometimes it was okay not to have answers, as long as we could move forward. She was also there with me, six months later, when we suddenly didn't see our next baby's heartbeat, and she helped me go forward with my future pregnancies.

Baby Angel #2, now named Noel

I didn't really acknowledge that I had given birth to Isla until after my second loss. I had treated the birth of my Baby Angel Girl, (whom we now have named Isla because seven years later, my living rainbow baby insisted that I name all of our babies), as a tragic event in my life that I had to overcome. I pushed forward, researched until my brain hurt, and then got pregnant again. When I lost that baby, now named Noel, I was left with even more devastation.

Noel came to me, I believe, to remind me that I could get pregnant and to trust my instincts, but nothing ever felt right during my pregnancy with her. I was late, but the pregnancy tests were never clear and direct like my other pregnancies. There was a faded pink line that got a little brighter every day, but I still knew in my heart that it wasn't right. I was told I was being paranoid, that this was past trauma worrying me, and that I should be elated and that I needed to focus on the good and not my past tragedy. But again, I just couldn't get excited, couldn't really celebrate.

We didn't tell anyone about my pregnancy with Noel. Isla's pregnancy and loss had been so public and so devastating. People we thought would be supportive, ended up making me feel worse about myself, my loss, and my grief. Many wanted me to just move on, and thought that getting pregnant again would do that. So, when Noel entered our life, I wasn't excited. I had this looming feeling of dread. I thought it was my grief and that I was protecting myself. I tried so hard to get excited, but I couldn't. It was like I truly knew that Noel was never meant to live in my arms. We did celebrate for one day, one, blissful 24 hours.

I had started spotting. I knew it was the end. We went in for an ultrasound, and the same, kind peritonologist was there to help us. And to our surprise, we saw a heartbeat! She was alive! Right there! She was small, but she was mighty! We cried tears of joy. We immediately went out to dinner in downtown L.A., celebrating that maybe, just maybe, I had been wrong about this pregnancy. After keeping things quiet for so long, Leif finally brought donuts into his work and told them he was going to be a dad again. After all, we were just one week shy of 12 weeks, the first trimester cut-off. We knew we had a long road ahead of us, but we were happy.

A week later, we went in for a check-up and another ultrasound to make sure everything was okay, and just like that, all my worries came true. No heartbeat. Somehow, I knew this was coming; I had expected it. I didn't cry. I wasn't shocked … I just went home and was truly quiet.

About an hour after the long, three-hour drive home from the perinatologist's office, I started to bleed heavily. I bled for weeks. I expected this, but it was different from Isla. My body held onto Noel, but it was also fighting with itself. I didn't want to drive to L.A. for a D&C, so I waited for three weeks. I lost Noel. Unlike Isla, I had tons of contractions, but never did it seem like a delivery. I had to go on. I went about my days. I remember having contractions in the middle of one of the classes I was taking and then sitting in a public bathroom stall, enduring the pain, hoping and not hoping that I would see her tiny little body. I never did.

Later, I learned that with a pregnancy that young, even with a heartbeat, my body probably absorbed Noel's. Doctors also told me that her death was probably due to, "Nature's way of fixing its mistakes." But it felt so real. *Why was my body broken? Why did God give me a baby, two babies, only to take them away? How could babies be mistakes?* I talked with counselors, friends who had lost children, and even friends with fertility problems.… *Why? Why? Why?*

I finally stopped asking, *Why?*, and realized that sometimes there isn't a why, except to make you a stronger, deeper person. And boy did I need to be that stronger person with the loss of my final baby, my boy.

Baby #3: Now named Tyler

After the birth of my rainbow baby, I honestly thought that our loss experiences were parts of a chapter in my life, a challenge that we overcame, a dark season to shape me into a better person. And while all this is true, pregnancy loss and life and death and birth are so much more complicated than a chapter in a story. My pregnancy with my rainbow baby and her birth had been so incredibly uncomplicated that it almost renewed my faith in this crazy journey of creating life. I am truly grateful for that period in my life. I don't know if I would still be on this earth if I had endured my son's loss without my rainbow baby's birth.

While I wish I could recount all the moments of Tyler's birth and death like Isla's and Noel's, I have to admit I really am not there, yet. Tyler's birth had so much trauma, and fear, and interventions, and seven long years of physical pain and trauma to my body that I still am processing it all. There are parts of that experience I have purposely blocked out for my own protection. I know there were times when I didn't know if I would survive his birth. I remember my living daughters, then five and two, arguing in the back seat, as we were driving to the hospital, as to whether I was okay and would live. They had such simple minds, there was not an ounce of anxiety in their voices. Mommy would survive, baby brother might not, but mommy would ... somehow, they knew that better than I did.

I have had many years of therapy, specialist visits, and lots of tests and surgeries and procedures and medications. While some of these moments I can really only relive in the safety of a therapist's chair, I do know a few things: birth is a miracle, it takes strong women to carry out the miracle of birth, even in the 21st century. We as humans do not have control over life and death and you cannot love a child into existence, because if that were the case, I would likely have several more than the five children I conceived.

I also know that I am a survivor. I am no longer mad or disgusted with my body that, for reasons no one knows, not even my God, couldn't bring all my babies to my arms. I knew after Tyler's birth that my body was telling me I was done giving birth. It couldn't handle one more intervention, one more loss, one more heartbreak. It took seven years for my heart to let go and listen to my body. Just this past year, my husband and I decided to end our quest for more children. We weren't really ready to stop trying, I don't know if we ever would be, but I knew I needed to shift my focus onto healing myself, and I have done just that.

I wish I could finish this tale with a happy ending. Before my son was born, I could have, but now I know better. Life isn't about happy endings. Trauma and struggles aren't just there to go through. The trauma and the struggles are also the beauty of life.

I now have two beautiful girls in my arms and three angels in heaven. Although the relationship I have with my God is messy and complicated, I do know I was meant to go through this journey. I know Isla and Noel were both there for me as I went through an incredibly fearful pregnancy that gradually transformed into one of the most empowering and enlightening times of my life: the birth of my second, earth-bound child. They helped me achieve goals I didn't even know I had of helping other women care for and breastfeed their babies; and they helped me define myself as a woman, a wife, and most importantly, as a mother.

I also know my son has truly shaped me into a person I didn't know could even exist. He showed me how strong I could be when I was at my absolute lowest. He showed me I could survive when I felt like no one wanted me to. And he helped show me that I had the capacity to love and care for others in a way that I had never even desired before.

Without these babies, I know I wouldn't be the person I am today. I miss them dearly, think of them often, and sometimes, still wonder why I never got to truly hold them. But I hold them in my soul, and they, forever, hold a piece of my heart, telling me to always follow my instincts, no matter how broken I may feel.

To my angels, who came into my life so briefly, but who will forever live as a part of me: I love you. I cherish you. Know that your mama is okay; she's a survivor. And to all the mothers and fathers of angels, no matter how old or young, please know, you are not alone.

Public Figures Share Their Personal Experiences To Help Others

Marquise and Morgan Goodwin –*Nineteen weeks – premature labor and human error*

Marquise Goodwin: "We experienced another traumatic event in our lives that we had to overcome, and it was tough [...] but I'll let Morgan go into detail about it."

Morgan: "Last season we found out we were pregnant during training camp and moving forward, that's why we were kind of keeping it like on the DL, like a secret, kind of keeping it a secret because I was afraid of a loss. Another loss. So I was going to hold out until I reached a certain point to where I really couldn't hide it anymore and then I also wanted to share it with you know our family and social media with *Goodwin SZN* [YouTube channel]. But unfortunately, it didn't go as planned. So in November, I experienced preterm labor and I was having contractions. I was in and out of the hospital and I was placed on bed rest. [...] I woke up at about three in the morning with some contractions that were really bad, and I rushed to the hospital. They were so bad that my water broke. And My doctor was like, 'Well, you have this permanent cerclage [...] there is no way that the baby can survive [...] from nineteen weeks all the way up until, you know, to give[ing] birth if the water is gone'. But

"We were carrying twin boys and basically, baby A's sac had ruptured when I was contracting. Um So, Baby B was still, you know, good but Baby A wasn't [...] So I had to have surgery to remove my stitch, my permanent cerclage, and they ended up rupturing that sac as well. And We were going to try to do a delayed delivery but it didn't end up not working out because they had made a mistake and ruptured my sac during the surgery—which we knew that this was a possibility, obviously, because they were sticking me with stuff in my stomach while I'm [was] under [...] anesthesia. [...] So that happened in November [...] and we're there trying to, you know, make it, you know, praying, and going through that but um, we're just taking it day by day."

Marquise: "Taking it day to day, and just comforting each other and doing different things to keep our minds busy and keep each other busy. Um, The dogs definitely keep our hands full, travelling [...], and um just showing each other love any time that we can. We appreciate y'all's support. We appreciate y'all for supporting us so much at this time."

Morgan: "Yeah, I finally had the courage to open up and talk about it, because I really didn't want to."

Marquise: "She didn't want to, but I think it, it'll probably be good for us. It helped last time: just, you know, moving past it and kind of finding our way. A lot of people reached out and that was cool. Uh, A lot of people sent us things last time and it just, it just helped to know how much we were loved by uh, either people we've come in contact with and even the people we haven't physically met. Um, Just to see how much you guys love and support us, we definitely appreciate that."

YouTube channel, GoodwinSZN. https://www.youtube.com/watch?v=FdLq6Zt4jl8

Two Little Lights

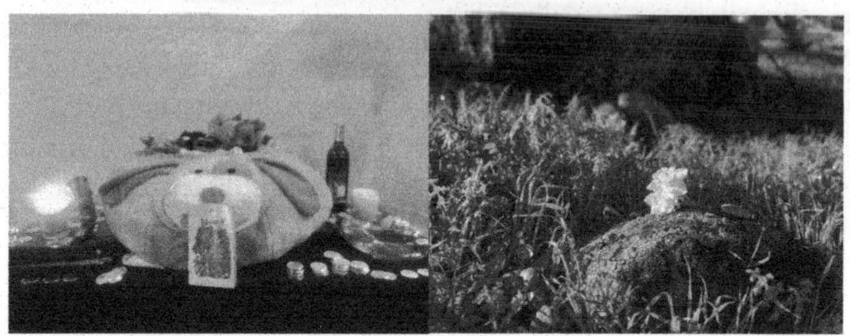

by Peter Wright

I read a story to you,
before you went away
Though you weren't there to hear it,
I read it anyway
There was a space that I made,
to keep the world at bay
a sacred space, just for you,
a place to say goodbye
the only way I knew how,
by spending all the time
I would never get to spend,
helping you to grow
Turning pages, one by one,
and reading from the glow
of candles lit for you,
and as the hours passed by
I honored you with precious things,
and silly things you'd love
told you of the man you were,
and what you would become
I knew you had to leave,
and I knew that I did too
and when the book was closed,

I put the cloth over you
I buried you with things,
I always thought I'd keep
but I wanted you to have them,
with you while you sleep
I wish you stayed a little longer,
but I did what I must
I bid you to the great existence,
surrounding all of us
And then the hardest thing, my son,
I took your little hand
said my first and last goodbye,
and watched you, as you ran

I carried a stone for you, my daughter,
so large my arms were full
over rough and far terrain,
but it was round and beautiful
And as your father, I should be strong,
so I showed you that I was
so you'd feel safe and loved beneath it,
and we'd know just where that was
We laid you beneath the tree,
that stays green all year round
We didn't know until you died,
exactly why that was
but it was waiting for you,
as it knew more than us
So it showed us through it's clover,
it was comfortable and soft
to tell us where to lay you,
when we sent you off
We set you in a sacred bowl,
where we'd poured our dreams to share
so when you slept behind our house,
we could be with you there
We gave you toys and candy,
and some stuffed animals too
and walked together slowly,

knowing what we had to do
We play there now sometimes with you,
ducking beneath the grass
and as your mother sits beside you,
time passes slowly by
She sings you songs in the wildflowers,
and sometimes, she cries
We'll always be here beside you,
and as your sister grows
when she plays beside your stone,
we think, somehow, she knows

Public Figures Share Their Personal Experiences To Help Others

Lily Allen – *Six months. Unknown/Undisclosed.*

"I went into early labour and they put a stitch in my cervix to try and stop that from developing, and that lasted for the best part of a week.

"The stitch broke and I went into full-blown labour and the baby was really, really small.

"And as I was delivering him, the doctors said, 'there was a pulse and now there no longer is.' The cord was wrapped around his neck and he was just too small."

"He was so small he actually got stuck halfway in and halfway out, so to speak, during the delivery, and because his skin wasn't fully formed they couldn't [use] forceps [to] pull him out."

"So there was a period of about 12 hours of lying there with him deceased in between my legs, which was incredibly [traumatic] […] I don't think I'll ever really recover from that."

https://www.thesun.co.uk/tvandshowbiz/7309636/lily-allen-womens-hour-tears-stillbirth/

"It was horrendous and something I would not wish on my worst enemy. It's something that I still haven't dealt with. I never will get over it. I have dealt with it, you know, as being at one with it. But it's not something that you get over.

"I held my child and it was really horrific and painful—one of the hardest things that can happen to a person.

"I nearly died. But I was numb and I didn't care. I'd just lost my baby and that is a reflection of how numb I was.

"I was overwhelmed by what an incredibly unlucky thing it was to happen, But I had [my husband] standing by my side, who I knew was going to be with me for the rest of my life."

https://www.eonline.com/news/531778/lily-allen-talks-devastating-still-birth-i-nearly-died-and-i-didn-t-care

You Were the Best Thing I Ever Knew I Needed, My Prince

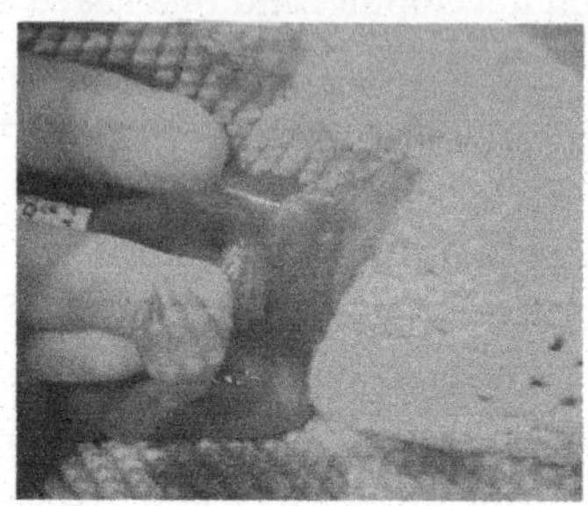

by Lauren Kirwin

I'm Oliver James' Mummy. Here is my story...

The beginning:

Finding out I was pregnant was the most unexpected surprise of my life; I'd only been in an official relationship for three months (with someone I'd known for years). It was the 3rd of January, 2016 when I found out I was expecting a little bundle of joy. Clear Blue said I was two to three weeks in, which apparently means five weeks. But anyway, about a week later, I was having major stomach pains and serious bleeding. Sorry to be graphic but it was clump after clump of new and old blood clots. It would be worrying for anyone, of course, so off to Accident and Emergency I went.

After waiting for about four hours, I got a bed. After another hour, I got seen and checked over. At that point, I was beyond being convinced everything was all right. The first words out of the doctor's mouth were, "Expect the worst; you've probably lost it!" He didn't examine me. A nurse came in again around an hour later. She then used the speculum to see if my cervix was open or closed. The good news was that it was closed, but just to be on the safe side, she sent me for a emergency scan. (How it's still an "emergency" scan four days later, I don't know!)

When arriving, I was petrified, obviously. In the room, I was told to lie on the bed. After using the ultrasound, they couldn't find any baby or heartbeat, but just to double check, they used the transvaginal (internal) ultrasound. She turned the screen and showed me my little baby bean for the first time; at six weeks and two days, I saw my baby's strong and healthy heartbeat! Of course, I sent everyone that knew about the pregnancy a picture and my scan!

On to the twelve-week scan:

There had been no problems at all since baby Bean's little mischievous act (making me worry like hell). He obviously wanted me to see him sooner rather than later! My boy's heart was still going strong, and seeing him bounce around on the screen just melted my usually ice-cold heart! He even seemed to give me a little wave! A couple of hours later, after showing close friends and family the scan photo, we announced it to the world on Facebook!

Of course, after seeing my Bean twice already, I couldn't wait any longer to find out if I was having a Prince or Princess. So, I booked an early gender scan and my little Bean was officially a Prince, mummy's little Prince! It was time to shop and get ready to spoil him like crazy (I even booked days off work so I could shop 'till I dropped)!

A few days later:

After a fun-filled few days buying half of the Disney Store's Dumbo merch and Disney baby clothes, I went for a trip to see my friend in Durham University and gave her the good news in person! After the chat and packing, it was time to bring her home for the holidays.... Never did I ever think that this trip would be the cause of seeing my boy's beautiful face too soon.

On the way home, we decided to stop off at Wetherby Services to get some food (I was eating for two of course!). When we pulled up to the roundabout, it was busy; cars were flying by. As it turned out, a car was also flying up behind us and BAM! straight into the back of us. The driver was on his phone, going 40 mph, approaching a busy roundabout! I had whiplash, abdominal bruising and swelling, a burn on my neck from the seatbelt, and a busted lip.

I had another emergency scan to check on my boy. Everything was fine; they said the fluid was a little low, but not to worry!

My boy's birth:

Suddenly, around a week after the crash, all was not fine. I'd been out during the day with friends, having a catch-up and a game of crazy golf. After getting home, I was absolutely done in, tired and drained after a full day of catching up. Around 9 p.m. I got a belly ache; I just passed it off as wind (I'd had a lot over the past few weeks), so it was time to get wrapped up in bed with a cup of tea, a Disney film, and a hot water bottle! Pure bliss!!! Everything was perfect.

On the 17th of April, 2016, at eighteen weeks and five days, I went out to play another round of mini golf. I had a lot of aches and pains but nothing more than what I had felt on other days, so we went home, got a cuppa' and a hot water bottle, and got in bed at around 8 P.M. I struggled to sleep that night and was up and down to the toilet until 11:30 P.M. As I went to wipe, I felt something odd between my legs. I thought I was dreaming. I put my hand there and felt something, so I got back in bed but brought a towel and placed it underneath me to make myself a little more covered and comfortable, as I knew in my heart what was coming. As I lay back down, I felt the urge to push and as we all know, it's not something we can stop.

At 12:20 A.M., my precious Oliver came into the world. Pure panic set in; I had no idea what to do. I tried to scream for help but nothing came out so I banged on the wall to my mum's bedroom. Still nothing. It took all my strength to scream for her. I could hear the shock and tiredness in her voice when she replied, "What's wrong?" "He's come out,'" I said. She said, "What? Who has?" Obviously she was still half asleep. After she came running into my room, the look on her face confirmed what I could only describe as a nightmare. My beautiful baby boy was now my very own angel.

My mum is a district nursing sister and, in that moment, she actually rang 911 instead of 999, a number she rings daily, and even she didn't know what was fully going on. While waiting for the ambulance, she had phoned the baby's daddy, who turned up just in time to follow the ambulance that came and took me to the hospital. The poor paramedic who picked Oliver up and cradled him and took great care told me his wife had gone through the same thing just weeks ago. I could see the pain in his eyes.

At the hospital, we went into a delivery room in the maternity ward and, yes, I could hear other babies but at that point, I was so withdrawn, I didn't really hear them. I was lucky enough to have a cuddle cot in the hospital and have Oliver with me through the whole two days I was in there.

After five tries to get a cannula in, and me being sick on the nurse, and two tries with a tablet to get the placenta to remove itself, and a pessary, I had to go to the operating theatre and be prepped at 9 A.M., before infection set in. I got delayed three times. I sent baby daddy home at 7 A.M. so he could sleep, but my mum was still with me. At 3:30 P.M., I was finally in the theatre. I was given the dreaded needle to numb my bottom half. I can tell you, it was painful. It got worse. I had a reaction to the injection and couldn't stop shaking.

Fast-forward:

The surgery was a success and the recovery was absolutely fine. After the recovery suite, I was sent back to the delivery room and it was time to tell our families and friends what had happened. I just did a copy and paste job of "Baby Oliver James was born sleeping this morning at 12:20 A.M.! My tiny little baby boy is now the brightest star in the sky." Replies started to flood in so I just turned my phone off.

Later that night, around 8 P.M., I was so hungry after not being allowed to eat anything apart from dry, cardboard hospital toast. My best friends came and brought me McDonald's: BEST MEAL EVER. At that point, everyone came and saw my beautiful boy; they gave him kisses, cuddles, and even sang to him.

After two days of antibiotics, checks, and signatures, I was allowed to go home. I held Oliver, kissed him, and took in every inch and feature. When I left the room, I was silent, and as soon as I got in the car, I cried my heart out, knowing I'd left him all alone. I couldn't forgive myself for leaving him. I still have nightmares about that day; counselors haven't helped.

Oliver stayed with me the whole time we were there, apart from when I had to go into surgery (the placenta just wouldn't come away by itself so it had to be removed). A post mortem was done: nothing was wrong with him. He was a perfect baby boy, just too small to survive! The rear-end crash caused my amniotic fluid to leak and that caused my waters to break and that caused early labor.

The funeral:

The one thing no parent should ever have to do is bury their child. Oliver was buried on the 12th of May, 2016, two days after my birthday. He was carried into the Church in a beautiful small wicker coffin while "The Circle of Life" from *The Lion King* was playing. During the service, I chose to have another song played, "You'll Be in My Heart" from *Tarzan*, a perfect fit for a perfect boy! After a very emotional service, we exited the Church to "He Lives in You" from *The Lion King 2* (a little Disney-mad if you didn't already realize, but all perfect songs.) We then made our way to his forever-bed. Close family and friends had a blue rose to place on his coffin after he was lowered. Everyone dropped their roses in but I just froze; I couldn't make myself stand over the hole where I was leaving my baby.

It was the best service I could ever have wanted and perfect for my little man. I couldn't believe how many people came to see my boy in his final resting place and to support me through that devastating time. I can't thank them enough!

Mummy loves you forever and always.

Forever, my Prince.

Public Figures Share Their Personal Experiences To Help Others

Chrissy Teigen – *Between 20 and 24 weeks. Pregnancy Complications.*

"We are shocked and in the kind of deep pain you only hear about, the kind of pain we've never felt before. We were never able to stop the bleeding and give our baby the fluids he needed, despite bags and bags of blood transfusions. It just wasn't enough.

"We never decide on our babies' names until the last possible moment after they're born, just before we leave the hospital. But we, for some reason, had started to call this little guy in my belly Jack. So he will always be Jack to us. Jack worked so hard to be a part of our little family, and he will be, forever.

"To our Jack - I'm so sorry that the first few moments of your life were met with so many complications, that we couldn't give you the home you needed to survive. We will always love you.

"Thank you to everyone who has been sending us positive energy, thoughts and prayers. We feel all of your love and truly appreciate you.

"We are so grateful for the life we have, for our wonderful babies Luna and Miles, for all the amazing things we've been able to experience. But everyday can't be full of sunshine. On this darkest of days, we will grieve, we will cry our eyes out. But we will hug and love each other harder and get through it."

Instagram https://www.instagram.com/p/CFyWQLWpJ3u/?utm_source=ig_embed&ig_rid=64dae76c-dda1-4b52-8244-d07902c-76c0d

26

Healing From Loss

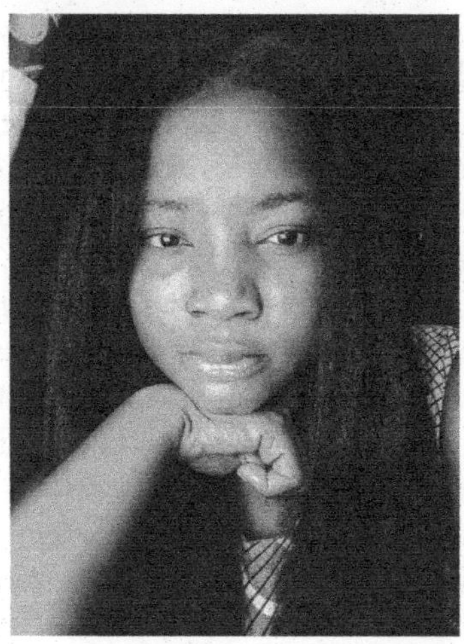

by Eze Modester

I am a mother of three angel daughters and I also have two living children (both boys) whom I love with all my strength. The youngest was a preemie born at 30 thirty weeks; he is currently nine years of age. I started experiencing loss after my two boys were born.

I had my first loss in October, 2017 at 23 weeks and 4 days. It all started one sad morning with painless bleeding, which intensified and consequently led to the premature birth of my baby girl at the hospital. My second loss was just like the previous one. It happened in May, 2019. I was 23 weeks and 3 days along. I had the same symptoms and I eventually lost her, too. My third loss was especially painful. I was 25 weeks and 5 days pregnant. It happened on February 6, 2020. I had the same symptoms as the first two times. I had even gotten a cerclage placed early on in the pregnancy to keep the baby in until delivery but my third little angel was not spared either.

Each loss brought me a great amount of pain but with the third loss, I became completely broken and totally shattered. Nobody seemed to understand me, neither family nor friends; perhaps they tried but didn't know how best to do it. At one point, my sister, in a bid to console me, told me that I shouldn't waste my tears on my dead babies because they are "Ọgbanje!" In this part of the world, when a woman continually experiences pregnancy loss, her babies are believed to be Ọgbanjes (children who die at birth and keep coming back to the family to be reborn several times). It is said that as a mother who experiences this, you are not expected to grieve; otherwise, such babies will keep coming back just to torment you. They die again and again, just to cause you pain. I was greatly disappointed that, in this age and time, such superstition is still believed.

The doctors and nurses were not caring, to say the least. At the delivery ward, where I lay with tears rolling down my cheeks after giving birth, the nurses and doctors chatted away with lovely smiles on their faces without taking into account my loss or pain. A doctor once told me, "Ma'am, I am so sorry for your loss but we can't prioritize your child over you; you are more important to us than the baby." After hearing those words, I only cried more and muttered silently in my heart, *Well, my babies are more important to me than me! You should have prioritized them over me.*

After all of my losses, I was never given the opportunity to hold them or see their faces. I even begged the nurses to take a picture of my baby but the matron bluntly refused.

I don't know if I will ever, ever try to get pregnant again because the truth is, I am afraid! The causes of my miscarriages are not yet diagnosed and I can't gamble with fate anymore.

I looked for ways to get back on my feet. I started exercising and losing weight which I have always wanted to do. I started reading more and more and I must confess, it has been really helpful.

My losses have taught me to be more compassionate towards people going through pain of any kind. If you are a mom or dad who has lost their precious angel and you happen to come across my story, I want you to know that you are loved, your angel is not taboo and you should be unapologetic when you talk about him or her. I am sending you hugs and prayers!

With love, Modester!

Public Figures Share Their Personal Experiences To Help Others

Katey Sagal – *Almost 8 months. Unknown/Undisclosed.*

> "It was a difficult thing; I lost a child at almost eight months, and… could not wrap my brain around it.
>
> "This is what they say about stillbirth, that 60 percent of it it's God's will, and there's no medical reason – and that's what I was told. And I just couldn't let go of the control of somehow, I had done something wrong.
>
> "Sometimes we have these little souls that come in and out of our lives, and their mission is complete."
>
> https://news.amomama.com/282804-married-with-childrens-katey-sagal-said.html

27

Jennifer's Story

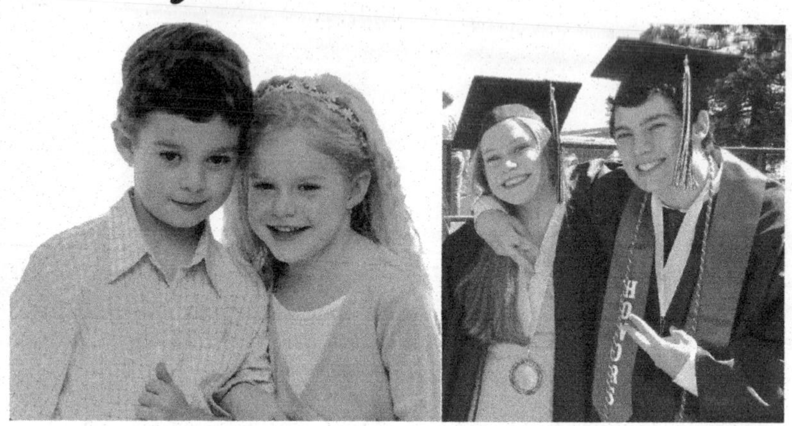

by Jennifer Coulter

It was 1995. I was 31 years old. My husband Craig and I had been married a little more than a year. We were on a six-month stay in New Zealand when we became pregnant. This was to be our first child and we were absolutely overjoyed, but I was feeling extremely sick, weak with a lot of headaches. I could not wait to go home to California. Once we got back, it took us a while to get settled into a house. I had to locate a doctor and wait for coverage. It turned out, this gap in my care made a huge difference to the way things played out, though I am grateful for the extra time I had with my unborn daughter.

Despite the fact that I thought she was going to be a boy, I was connected to her from the very beginning. I remember one special moment I had with her. I was lying alone in my bed with my hands on my tummy, telling her how much I loved her. I could feel it so strongly in my heart that it hurt. What happened next was utterly amazing. I could feel her pressing into my hand. The pattern was deliberate, a rhythmic motion. It felt like her little hand was pressing into my hand and she did this repeatedly five or six times. By now, I was used to the kicks, twists, and turns, but this was not that. This was her saying, "I love you mama. I am here and I feel your love!"

My first check-up after returning to California was my first experience with a state medical doctor. During this appointment, he did not examine me at all; he only asked me some basic questions, filled out some paperwork and headed towards the door. I then asked him, "Is it normal for my stomach to feel so tight?" He stopped and came back in. He examined my large tummy and he asked me to meet him at the room down the hall for an ultrasound. There, the look on his face was terrifying. I could tell that he was surprised. At first, he thought I could have a tear or leak, or, worst-case scenario, it was Potter Syndrome. He explained that I had no amniotic fluid and sent me home for bedrest for three days to see if things would change. They did not. He made an appointment for another ultrasound at the hospital. Back in 1995, ultrasounds were, well, not nearly as sharp they are now.

I went to the appointment by myself. I was terrified. They asked me if I would mind if a visiting doctor sat in on the ultrasound. This doctor was only there for that one day and it turned out his doctoral thesis was on Potter Syndrome. I could not believe my luck! Now I had faith that I could trust their findings. The ultrasound lasted two hours. The intensity of having those two doctors and others popping in to consult, made me realize they knew they had my baby's life in their hands. They had to find, or not find, kidneys. They could not locate them. It took two hours of using every angle and exhausting all possibilities. That little black and white monitor just looked like a bunch of white dots to me. In the end, they were confident with their diagnosis.

I was given a choice: they would induce delivery, or I could carry her full-term and go into labor normally. Either way, the outcome would be the same; she would not survive. I had a huge decision to make.

If I were to deliver her prematurely, then I had to be 100% certain the diagnosis was correct and that she could not survive on her own. I was told due to the medicines they use when they induce labor, that she would not survive it, regardless of her diagnosis.

I seriously contemplated carrying her to full-term but every time I tried to picture it, I knew I could not do it. I was already so bonded with her. Every day, having her growing inside me, being perfectly fine while she was in the safety of my womb, becoming more and more attached and all the while knowing we would lose her; I could not imagine spending eight more weeks knowing she could not live. I did not rush to my decision. I prayed a lot.

My husband did not know what to do. He told me that he would be behind me all the way, whatever I decided. I discovered that while I could talk to my friends and family, ultimately this was a decision only I could make. I knew that I had to be sure, as I did not want to have any doubts or regrets for this terrible decision.

At seven months pregnant, we had already set up the crib and began setting up the nursery, before we received that heartbreaking diagnosis. I could not go in there; it hurt too much. I woke up one morning and the answer was clear. I knew it would only become more difficult, and time would not be my friend. I had to just take the step and have them induce me for delivery.

Our daughter died of Potters Syndrome. I delivered her at 32 weeks.

Because of the abortion policies back then, I had to go to a state hospital. In the hospital, I felt like a fragile piece of glass that at any moment, if I were not careful, would shatter into a thousand shards. A few friends and family wanted to come to the hospital, but I knew I would break if I had to see their sadness and my despair reflected in their eyes. I told them I was sorry, but I could not have visitors. All I needed was my husband and I would be fine. My mother was very hurt by my decision and in the end, I allowed her to come in.

I floated in little glass bubbles for hours and hours. I am not sure how long it was. But then, there she was. They whisked her away before I could touch her or hold her. They promised they would bring her back and they did. It was a very strange thing to finally hold my baby. So many things ran through my mind. There really are no words to properly describe it.

They put me in a room to recover by myself for a little while. I must have passed out, because the next thing I knew, I was in a different room in the general ward. I was told I was sharing a room with an older lady who was recovering from surgery. You see, with cases like mine, they do not put you in the maternity ward. They say it is hard on the grieving mothers to hear babies crying and the happy sounds of new mothers, fathers, and visitors with their precious bundles of joy.

I was extremely upset. I wanted to scream! I wanted to shout! I wanted to cry. But I felt I could not. This poor woman next to me, with the curtain drawn between our beds, was just a thin piece of fabric away. I tried to hold it in, but I just could not any longer. I needed to cry. I told them I needed my own room; I could not stay there. I knew I could not go through this quietly while constantly worrying about people through shared curtains. Of course, being in a state hospital, this was out of the question. It was a living nightmare; I needed to scream or I would burst!

Craig tried as hard as he could, but it seemed nothing was going to get me out of this microscopic room. He did not even try to talk me out of it; he could see the desperation on my face. I finally said, "I can't walk but I have no choice. Get me out of here!" My poor husband went to the staff and explained, "She desperately wants to leave. We need a wheelchair." The shocked nurses told him that I was not allowed to leave. He came back into the room and told me what they said. Now I was at my wits end. I said, "Just watch me!" Craig found me a wheelchair himself and we just left. It was dark and cold at 11:30 p.m. on March 23 and he wheeled me right out of that god-awful place. My own bed was all I wanted. After that, everything was a blur.

A few days later, I received a phone call from the hospital. The man on the phone asked me what I wanted to do with the baby. I was so beside myself with grief, I did not know what he meant. *What is he talking about?*

I had not even thought about it. I do not know why, but I asked him, "Do you take care of the baby or do I take care of the baby?" And the man on the phone simply said, "We can take care of the baby." He made it sound so easy, so I said, "OK. Do that."

Looking back, I still get angry that not one person, family, friend, or social worker, had offered to go over this necessary and ugly detail with us. I was in no position to be making that decision. Why hadn't anyone asked me, or told me that this is not what I should do?

A week or two went by and I woke up one day from a deep sleep ... I sat straight up. *Where is my baby?* I did not know where she was! I was practically hysterical. *Oh my God! What did I do?!* I was panicked, completely beside myself. I had to find my baby! *What did they do with her? What was I thinking? Why didn't somebody intervene and help me with all of this?* I was screaming, "Where is my baby?!" I was all alone, again, trying to figure out what to do and trying to calm myself down.

I called the hospital right away and explained the situation. A kind person checked into it and got back to me in a few hours. I was told they had my baby and they just needed to know where to transfer her. I was so relieved! I located a mortuary and set up arrangements to have a graveside burial. On the day of the funeral, I was doing my best to stay in control. I was not going to break down. About an hour before the funeral, my mother called and asked me who would be attending the funeral. We got into a little tiff about the fact that my nephew would be attending. She said in an irritated voice, "He doesn't care about the baby, he only wants a reason to get out of school." When she said that, I thought to myself, *Oh no, not again!* I told her, "He cares about me and my baby. He came over and helped set up the crib in the nursery." I do not remember what she said after that, but by the tone of her voice, I knew anything else she said would push me over the edge. My survival instincts kicked in and I hung up the phone.

I picked the phone back up to call my husband and tell him what she said but I could still hear her; she was still ranting! She did not even know I had hung up. I quietly put the receiver back down. I could not take it, not right before my baby's funeral. I had to keep myself together.

We were at the cemetery, graveside. The casket was so small.... The minister was waiting, everyone was waiting. My brother was agitated, trying to figure out where my mother was. (Nobody had cell phones yet.) He kept saying, "She will be here, of course she will be here. Let's just give her a few more minutes." But I had a bad feeling. *Would she really do this? Could she not see past herself and understand that I could not take her drama? Not now, not today!*

We waited for fifteen minutes ... I knew she was not going to show up. I had hung up on her after all; maybe she thought she was the victim here. She would show me; she would not come to my baby's funeral. She would force me to explain to everyone why my own mother would not show up to such an important event. I could not believe she would do this to me. Everyone asked me where she was, was she okay? I chose to explain what had taken place and let them do with it what they wanted. I had no shame. Ultimately, those that knew my mother understood; those that did not, oh well, what could I do?

Sadly, at the wake, I spent a good deal of time having to explain her absence and feeling judged. It was so unfair, that day of all days. We only had that small window of time to receive the gifts of support and condolences. It would have been nice to focus on that important ceremony to give us closure and yet, that was not what happened. I could have lied and said she had come down with a migraine and could not come, but that is not who I am. I can't lie. That was the last time I spoke to my mother for three years.

We eventually reconciled, only to become estranged again for another two years. As good wine ages with time, good people do also. Time heals a lot of wounds. When it was my mother's time to leave this earth, she was ready and at peace. She died of pancreatic cancer in 2017.

After the funeral, I was left completely devastated. I could not eat or do anything. I could only stare at the TV with the volume muted. Sleep took on a whole new meaning. I would drift in and out, day and night. I cried all the time. I would wake up and remember what had happened and I would just cry out, "My baby! My baby!" I was inconsolable. This went on for weeks and then months. I could not see how I was ever going to cope.

Until, one day, I dragged myself out of bed. I was sitting alone, as usual, on the couch, looking out the window. It did not take long for me to start crying again but this time I was angrier. I cried out to God, "Why? Why?" I was praying and asking God to help me. My despair was so deep. I had been grieving for so long that I could not think of anything beyond this huge devastation and the agony of life moving forward. I did not know how much more of this I could take. I was mad!

Then, suddenly, something happened. A little movie started playing inside my head. Instantly, I was transfixed. I was entranced, looking outside at a big green lawn. It was a warm day. Then, right in front of me, this little boy with dark brown hair and big brown eyes was running around and around in circles with his arms flapping out from his sides like he was flying, throwing his head back while giggling and laughing! He was filled with the kind of joy that you get from simply running barefoot in the grass. He was beautiful! I was captivated.

And then, that was it; it was over. As fast as it overtook me, it was gone. I could not believe it. I had just been blessed with a vision. I knew that little boy was going to be my son one day! I sat there forever, reliving each precious second. I did not want to forget that face, his eyes, his brown hair, the sound of his laughter. It was so real!

After that, a calmness fell over me I had not felt before. I was certain that everything was going to be OK. I prayed and I thanked God for blessing me. I did not know then that over the next three years, I would go on to lose three more precious babies. This vision, this tiny peek into the future, is what got me through the tough times ahead.

When I looked back at the delivery of my first baby, I realized that there were some things I did not pay any attention to at the time but made sense later. Right when I delivered her, I asked the nurses, "Is it a boy? Is it a boy?" I remember seeing their confused faces as they were looking at my baby. They looked at each other and then one said, almost hesitantly, "Yes, yes. It's a boy." I said, "I knew it!" *I always knew I would have a boy first.*

When I was holding her, I was looking over her body as only a mother would. Something was not right; there was no sign of her being a boy or a girl. In the moment, I panicked. Then I thought, *What are you doing? Just hold your baby while you can.*

Because they told us she was a boy, we named her Kyle. Her middle name was to be John, after Craig's father who died when he was in high school. About two months later, when we received the autopsy report, we got the after-shock. They told us that he was a girl! They had found ovaries. The diagnosis has been confirmed; Potter syndrome with ambiguous genitalia; it explained why the nurses did not know what to say and why I did not see anything during my brief, cursory exploration.

We could not believe such a thing could happen. *What do we do now?* The headstone had already been ordered. For over two months, we had been saying, "He," and, "Him" ... "Kyle". After a few days, we realized we could add another "e" on the end and we named her Kylee J. I did not want to have to tell everyone but I could not keep calling her "him." So, we decided to tell our inner circle what happened. At this point, I was tired of explaining everything. I wanted life to be normal again.

Luckily, I did not have to return to work right away. I just stayed home and grieved for six months. When I was ready to go back to work, I contacted my old employer and they put me on assignment. As luck would have it, the manager of the large apartment community was set to go on maternity leave, so getting back to work was nice at first, to get my mind off things. But it turned into a nightmare.

As a lot of the managers do, the lady I was temporarily replacing lived in the community. Almost daily, she would come to the office to show off her baby. I was happy for her and I felt guilty for not wanting to join in with all the "ooohs" and "awws." Instead, I would quietly slip out of the office and go for a walk. One day, she stayed an exceptionally long time, going on and on, telling the whole office about all the finer details of new motherhood. I could not take it; I was so careful to even avoid the baby aisle at the grocery store and yet, there I was, held hostage at my desk. I had to leave the room. It was then that she realized what was happening. She had not thought of it before. She apologized profusely. She felt so bad, which made me feel bad. It was just my rotten luck to get this particular assignment.

Our second precious baby was with us for 18 weeks. I had just gone out and purchased a whole new maternity wardrobe. Luckily, I had not worn them and since I had not removed the tags, Craig was able to make the return. I had been feeling like something was not right. I kept trying to describe how I was feeling and for several weeks I could not put my finger on it. One night, I told Craig, "I think I finally figured it out,; I just do not feel pregnant anymore." The next day, I went to the doctor and they found no heartbeat. They measured the fetus and told me the baby had died two weeks prior. There is a lesson here: never doubt a mother's intuition. In my case, it would not have mattered. But it is a true testament to our ability to know.

They sent me home only to return the next day for a procedure to prepare me for the surgery to take place on the following day. The next two days were tough. I remember lying in the bath, holding my tummy, crying. Being very thin, I was showing a nice baby bump. It is hard to explain, knowing that your baby has passed, and yet, there you are, carrying it. Another time in life when there are no words to fully describe what I was feeling.

That type of surgery was also emotionally difficult. I took that loss hard, but I reminded myself: I had my gift. I had my vision. I knew one day I would have a son! I was strong and even though I experienced a deep grief, it did not interfere with my job or my life. I just kept on having faith. Craig and I put our energies into our very first house.

I am not sure how long it was, but soon after, number three came along. This wee one was with us for 16 weeks. Then, same as before: no heartbeat. Rinse and repeat; same two days of horror and same surgery. Sadly, I was getting familiar with this process. I took it on the chin and barely cried at all. After all, I had my secret weapons. I had my faith, and my bestowed vision.

It had been nearly three years since we lost Kylee, and I was pregnant yet again, for a fourth time! At ten weeks, I suffered a spontaneous miscarriage when I was at home alone. This was before cell phones were common, and I had no way to call my husband. I called my best friend and she stayed on the phone with me as I went through it. It was very painful, but I dealt with it on my own. I was urged to go right to the hospital. But I knew better. I had faith in myself and my knowing. I'd had enough of hospitals. I called my doctor and made an appointment for the next day. Then

I waited for Craig to come home. I do not recall crying, not even one tear. I had my special gift to keep me strong. I was firm in my faith.

By now, after losing four babies, I was sure I knew why. No doctor would confirm it; after all, they had some liability. When I was 23 years old, I battled a severe case of Graves' disease. I tried medication therapy for nearly a year: 14 pills every day. I was even on heart medication. I could barely hold down my job. When it was obvious the medicine was only making me sicker, I was given a round of radioactive iodine. These days, you simply take a pill, but back then, they used a heavy, lead container that contained a beaker held firmly in place with foam, so it didn't touch the sides.

The doctor covered himself with heavy equipment to block the radiation. Then he handed me a plastic straw and said, "Here, drink it." The beaker was half full of what they called a "nuclear cocktail." He kept adding water to the beaker and I kept having to drink it. I wanted to vomit but I had to keep drinking. After two months, they gave me a second round of radiation.

It was hard; I was young and terribly sick for three years. They told me I could not get pregnant for at least a year after the treatments. They said it damages the eggs and they did not know how far and deep the damage would go. I recently read that they do not give this treatment to women under 30. I know why. I also believe these same treatments caused me to have four, non-cancerous breast tumors and two tumors on my thyroid. When Craig and I started to become serious, I told him I did not know if I could ever have children. I had to be upfront and honest. He said he did not care; he loved me anyway.

That special day arrived when I was 35. We found out we were pregnant for the fifth time. I was positively glowing the whole time I was pregnant with Ryan. Everyone was worried – but I was not. I knew everything was going to be OK and I told everybody not to worry. We were given a wonderful baby shower filled with a lot of love! I was peaceful through the entire pregnancy. Craig and I had started a business a few year earlier, so I prepared for my departure and replacement. All was good. All was perfect!

Ryan Pierce arrived in the world March 17, 1999. Seven pounds of perfect! He had brown hair and big, beautiful, brown eyes! I had seen that face before.

The delivery, however, was extremely difficult. We almost lost him. He became stuck and it was very intense. It is never good when you see fear on your doctor's face. My small frame was the cause. I had severe tearing and had to stay in the hospital for several days. Due to the long time that he was stuck, he had breathing problems and had to be in the NICU for five days. It was awful and I just wanted to bring our beautiful boy home, but again, I knew everything was going to be OK.

I will never forget the first day we brought him home. We could not take our eyes off him! We stared at him for what seem like forever. Then we looked at each other and said, "Now what?" After everything we had been through, we had no clue what to do next! We still laugh about that to this day!

Months went by. He was a fussy boy. Night was day, day was night; with no family to help us, it was hard. I even missed my check-up with the OB. When I went for my first visit at 14 weeks, I opted for an IUD. I finally had my sweet gift; I could not go through that again. My husband was disappointed but supportive.

Time passed and I was completely absorbed and deeply in love with my baby boy. I was not paying attention to the calendar, though I had noticed I was starting to put on weight. Then there was the argument. Craig and I only have fights like that when I am pregnant and we both knew it. He said to me, "If I did not know any better, I would swear you were pregnant!" We stopped and stared each other. We quietly dropped the subject and went to our separate corners. You recognize the truth when you hear it, so I quickly left to get a test. I showed him the test and without saying anything, we went through the motions. We had been through this so many times already.

The test was positive. We were pregnant with our sixth child! We were speechless. *How could this be?* As the enormity of the situation flooded over us, we each had quite different reactions. I threw the test across the room, dropped to the floor, and started bawling. He began jumping up and down, whooping and hollering and running all around the house! He ran out through the garage, into the street, and back to the house again! I have never seen a reaction like that from him. He was elated! I was very entertained by his reaction and of course, I was extremely happy! Though I must admit, I was baffled as to how this actually happened.

The next day we went to the doctor. They did the ultrasound but instead of seeing a little fuzzy peanut, we saw a fully formed baby! There she was, waving at us with her fully formed hand and five fingers, "Hi mom! Hi Dad! I've been waiting for you to figure out I'm here!" We were stunned. I was already well into the second trimester, and I didn't even know it!

We walked out of the office in a daze. There we were, almost five months pregnant, with an infant in a stroller, sitting on a park bench trying to wrap our brains around what the doctor had just told us. We were going to have another baby … and very soon. I often wonder how much longer it would have taken us to figure it out, if it had not been for that argument.

The next few months went by extremely fast. We decided to buy a more kid-friendly house. I was very pregnant, with an infant baby, packing, unpacking, and buying and selling houses. One day, I was walking through the new house with the cleaners. My legs started to feel heavy and I quickly found I could no longer walk. Being mothers themselves, they said, "Girl, you're going into labor!" I said, "No way. I'm not due for two more months!"

We raced to the hospital, ignoring stop signs and several red lights. I was going into hard labor that fast! As soon as I got there, they had to quickly discern through blood tests whether to stop the labor or to let it continue. The blood test showed high white blood cells which meant the IUD had become infected and I had to deliver her right away! The next thing I knew, I was holding a beautiful baby girl! She weighed exactly five pounds. Gabrielle Rose surprised us on December 20, 1999. She was gorgeous with her strawberry blonde hair. She was tiny but healthy. She was in the NICU for two weeks. A few days after she was delivered, her white blood cell count was practically nonexistent. The doctors prepared us for the worst. They said she might not make it. She had no protection even against herself! After three days, the treatments finally worked and she bounced back. That was one hell of a Christmas. I was going back and forth between the hospital and home to take care of Ryan.

I always laugh when I think about going into the NICU; the nurses would offer me guidance and assistance as they do for newborns. I would always say, laughing, "It's OK. I have one just like this at home!" Countless times over the years, I would see that same reaction: eyes wide, mouth open. Ryan was nine months and three days old when Gabby was born. Our little Irish twins! Even though Gabby was premature, she suffered no repercussions. She and her brother would learn and grow together at the same pace. Inseparable. They were very bright children and were high achievers in school.

My story does not end there. As I approach my 56th birthday, I look back over my life in amazement. I had one more missing piece of the puzzle yet to fall into place. It would take me several more years to figure it out. The way things played out was certainly interesting and we had some unexpected outcomes.

All my life I had thought I would have twins. At each ultrasound, I would always ask, "Is it twins?" Each time I would be disappointed, just shaking my head. You see, I had this picture in my head, another snippet of the future. I could see a boy and a girl standing side-by-side at graduation, in a full cap and gown. I was so sure I would have twins. Although Ryan and Gabrielle were close in age, the way the school system is in America, they would be in different grades; I could not understand how my vision had been wrong. I had no worries though, we had two beautiful children and I was lucky to be a full-time, stay-at-home mother. Life was good.

In 2003, out of the blue, someone placed an offer to buy our business and our house! We were not looking for this opportunity, but we decided to seize the moment and go for it. We moved to New Zealand to raise the children around our wonderful large family there.

The kids started school, as they do in New Zealand, the day after their fifth birthday, even if it is on a Thursday! The system is quite different there; the first three years is a kind of filtering process. It was explained to me that this is because the children are entering school at different times throughout the school year. Some are pushed forward; some may linger depending on their needs and when they arrived. This would prove to be an important factor that would lay the groundwork for the surprise that was to come.

We lived in New Zealand for three years. I became terribly ill and wanted to move back to California. We managed to re-immigrate ourselves and settled in. When we enrolled the kids in school, they put Ryan in second grade. He had already done most of the 2nd grade schoolwork in New Zealand, but we felt it was good for him to be with kids his own age. Gabby missed the cut-off by only ten days and they insisted on putting her in first grade. I explained that she had already nearly completed the second grade. During the second week of school, they tested her. She breezed through the first-grade curriculum and easily worked through the second-grade book. We were not surprised when her teacher bumped her up to the second grade, where she belonged. We were so relieved the children would not be struggling in school and could use their energy to acclimate to a different country. It was a big change for them. Three years is a long time for small children; they had even developed New Zealand accents!

The next year, when they were in third grade, it finally clicked in my head. I do not know why I did not think of it sooner! This meant that they would be graduating high school together! Side-by-side!

And so, they did, full cap and gown with honors. I had misinterpreted my vision. When I "saw" them, I had assumed they were twins. Who would ever guess it would take all those twists and turns to work out the way it did? My "knowing," the picture I had held in my mind of the two teens graduating together, was correct after all. I could not get over it! I felt validated. Life is amazing!

Ryan and Gabby are now both in their fourth year at the University of Nevada, Reno, living together as roommates. I remind them all the time that there is something special about them and the way they were born. And no matter what, to always have each other's back.

During my losses, I felt all alone, isolated from everyone. Craig worked a lot and was also bereaved, and he was as lost as I was. During hard times like these, a girl really needs her mom, but I did not have mine. Early on, I noticed most people would become uncomfortable if I mentioned my lost babies. Nodding heads and sympathetic words. I never wanted to make anyone uncomfortable, so I stopped talking about it. Cards, flowers, and casseroles are nice, but support was what I needed.

Death is such a sensitive subject; and when it is the death of a baby, it is even harder for people to relate to. They just do not know what to say. Heck, I went through it and I don't know what the magic words are. It is hard to know what the future will hold. Some days I feel tired, weak, beaten down, heavy with the burden from of all the ancient grief. For me, it does not go away. It has molded me into who I am today. Other times, I feel strong because I know I can handle anything. I have trust and faith in myself. I have conquered. When I look at myself in the mirror, I see a battle-torn warrior with deep scars, and wounds that I fear will never heal. My badge of honor is my faith.

Time is such a peculiar thing. Hindsight brings its own unique perspective that you learn from. I was blessed to receive snippets of hope. Without them, I do not know how I would have managed. If you have faith and you hold onto your beliefs, you can recognize and receive special gifts, too. But I find that you have to be open and ask to receive them. Everyone reacts differently when they are faced with the grieving process. Instead of looking to others to help us to feel better, we need to look within ourselves for inner strength. Maybe that is done through prayer, meditation, or journaling, or having the courage to find a support group that will understand. I hope sharing my story will help others. I believe, with all my heart, that we are not alone after all, even when we feel like we are. We have our own personal army on the other side, looking out for us. We just need to trust and be true to ourselves. Thank you for reading my story. It is my little life, my little truths.

If you are grieving, I wish for you to seek peace. If you know someone that is suffering, just remind them often how much they are loved.

Public Figures Share Their Personal Experiences To Help Others

Jackie Kennedy – *Eight months. Unknown/Undisclosed.*

"Jackie had already suffered one miscarriage in 1955 when she fell pregnant for the second time, and she knew carrying the child to term would be no easy task.

"Due in September of 1956, Jackie made it past the three-month mark – the stage where she miscarried the first time – through her second trimester and into the third before things went wrong.

"While JFK was away with friends cruising the Mediterranean on a yacht, Jackie's pregnancy came to an abrupt and heartbreaking end.

"She woke on the morning of 23 August 1956 bleeding heavily. Not long after, Jackie delivered their first child, a daughter Jackie named Arabella. She was stillborn.

According to reports, Jackie never officially named her first daughter, nor does the name 'Arabella' appear on any formal documents or in any written records.

"However, those closest to Jackie have claimed time and again that the former First Lady referred to her stillborn child by that name as she mourned in the months following the traumatic delivery. [...]

"Though only two of her children survived past infancy, Jackie reportedly viewed all of her pregnancies with the same love and devotion.

"When editing a book written by her friend, historian Arthur Schlesinger, Jackie confirmed that she and JFK had 'five children in ten years.'"

The tragic tale of Jackie Kennedy's firstborn daughter by Maddison Leach 2020

https://honey.nine.com.au/latest/jackie-kennedy-firstborn-daughter/2146cbcd-65c6-4497-8a6e-9215f2af2f08

28

My Sweet Althea

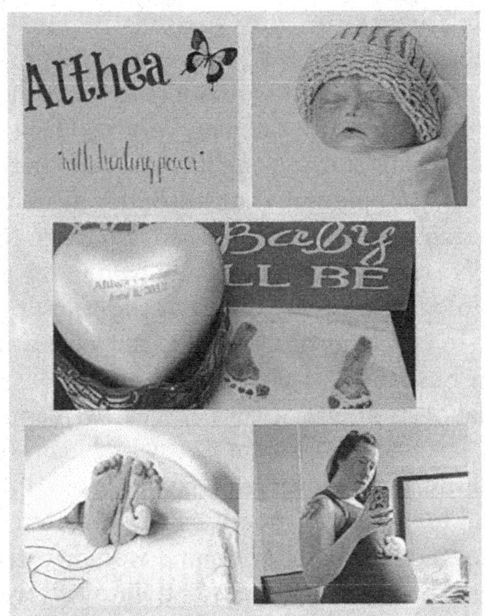

by Kelsey Kirkpatrick

My princess was born sleeping June 8, 2018. I woke up on the 6th at 32 weeks pregnant, excited for my ultrasound and to see my beautiful little girl.

I walk into the room and recline on the table. As I look at the screen and see her, my heart swells with love. Then the three words that continue to haunt me were spoken, "There's no heartbeat." Just like that; no emotion as she continues on with her measurements. She says nothing else, not even a few words of sympathy. At first I think it's a sick joke. She doesn't seem sincere. Then it hits me; she is serious.

Just then, my mom opens the door and walks in and I start crying. My mom (who has had multiple miscarriages) immediately understands what is going on. I tell her what the technician said. My mom is holding me ... then the tech asks if I want some ultrasound pictures. My mom answers for me, "You know what? Print some pictures and I will take them 'til she is ready." The lady looks at my mom and says, "I wasn't asking you, I was asking her." I remember her words and how cold she seemed to this day!

They take me to a room and tell me to wait for my doctor. I had already called my husband, telling him to come to the hospital. I don't even remember how that conversation went. I was in shock; the walls were closing in and my whole world was crashing around me. After my dad and husband get there, my doctor comes in. Everyone is crying around me and I am just sitting there.

My doctor tells me that I should deliver vaginally to help with future deliveries. I nod and agree that I would like to try it that way. I head to labor and delivery. They have to soften my cervix so I take a pill every four hours for a day and a half. Thursday night comes and they break my water at 8 P.M. and give me the epidural. I am still barely dilated so they send my husband home because nothing is supposed to happen that night.

Four A.M. rolls around and I am feeling pain in my pelvic area. They call the anesthesiologist to up my dose but the pain doesn't go away, so the nurse decides to check my progress. She can feel my little girl's head. I am told to call my husband and tell him it is time...

I went into labor at 4:59 A.M. and Althea Iwanlani Kirkpatrick was born at 5:05 A.M. She was 6 lbs. 6oz. at 32 weeks. No one spoke as she was born into a world she would never see.

I wanted to try for another as soon as I could, so, after my first period, the OBGYN gave us the okay to try again. I wouldn't suggest this for everyone since everyone heals and copes in their own way. My way was to move forward, to have something to look forward to!

September rolls around, only three months after my loss, and I see the two lines. I'm pregnant again! Cue the panic button. I can't help but worry, *what if I lose this one, too*?

I went to my first OBGYN appointment and they gave me an ultrasound – just one of so many more! My doctor also wanted me to go to a high-risk specialist at the same time so we could monitor everything even more. My high-risk doctor found out that I have something called Antiphospholipid Antibody Syndrome, a disorder in which the immune system mistakenly attacks normal proteins in the blood. Antiphospholipid syndrome can cause blood clots to form within the arteries, veins, and organs. It can also cause miscarriage and stillbirth. That was how I found out what caused my first baby to be stillborn.

To prevent this from happening again, my doctor had me give myself a shot of blood thinner every day 'til I delivered. I noticed how much better I felt. With my first, I was so sick the whole pregnancy! I couldn't stop puking and I had pre-eclampsia along with other issues. With this pregnancy, I barely ever felt pregnant. It was such an easy pregnancy, which scared me even more! We took the DNA tests to make sure nothing else would be wrong and at the same time to figure out the gender even sooner. We were having another girl! After 29 weeks, I had ultrasounds every other week and non-stress tests twice a week. At 32 weeks, ultrasounds switched to every week until I was at 35 weeks and 5 days, when they scheduled my induction.

We went in on April 11 at 6:30 p.m. to get the medicine inserted that would soften my cervix overnight. The next morning at 10 a.m., after I ate and showered, my doctor started me on Pitocin. She joked that she was off work at five o'clock so my daughter had better come before that.

Finally, I start feeling the contractions. I do have a high pain tolerance, but we are trying to get the epidural and the nurse keeps saying she is waiting for "active labor."

Finally, I tell her, "I'm in active labor! Get me the epidural now!" My body won't do anything without it. I have control issues and it helps me relax and hurries the process. We learned this with our first one.

At 3:50 p.m., the epidural is in and I can totally feel it. I'm feeling pressure at 4 p.m. I tell the nurse, "She is ready."

"You were just dilated to a 6, so I doubt it."

I make her check and she says, "Oh! I feel the head. She is a Q-tip, too. No hair!" She calls my doctor and the NICU (she was a month early) and I can feel my daughter trying to push her way out. So, there I am waiting for my doctor to show up and squeezing my legs together. At 4:15 p.m., she shows up and starts getting ready. At 4:20, they put my legs up and I can feel my daughter kicking off of me. I'm laughing and everyone else is laughing and my doctor turns around and Whoosh! my daughter birthed herself at 6lbs 12oz. I didn't push once.

With my first, the room was so quiet and sad ... with my rainbow unicorn, we were laughing the whole time. My Aulora Vanita is now almost a year-and-a-half and is the light at the end of the tunnel. She has helped me in more ways than I can count. But not a day goes by that I don't miss my angel, Althea.

Just know that if you are going through a loss, you are not alone! There are amazing groups on Facebook where you can connect with other loss parents who will help you through it. It is two years after my loss and I still find myself crying ... and that is totally okay. You are allowed to grieve forever. If you need a song to listen to that will help the tears come, "Winter Bear" by Colby Grant is an amazing one. I listen to it when I want to feel closer to my angel.

Public Figures Share Their Personal Experiences To Help Others

Keanu Reeves – *Eight months. Unknown/Undisclosed.*

> "... for the character and in life, it's about the love of the person you're grieving for, and any time you can keep company with that fire, it is warm. I absolutely relate to that, and I don't think you ever work through it. Grief and loss, those are things that don't ever go away. They stay with you [...] It's always with you, but like an ebb and flow,"
>
> https://www.theguardian.com/film/2019/may/18/keanu-reeves-grief-loss--bill-ted-john-wick-actor-tragedy

"Grief changes shape, but it never ends. People have a misconception that you can deal with it and say, 'It's gone, and I'm better.' They're wrong. When the people you love are gone, you're alone.

"I miss being a part of their lives and them being part of mine. I wonder what the present would be like if they were here – what we might have done together. I miss all the great things that will never be.

"All you can do is hope that grief will be transformed and, instead of feeling pain and confusion you will be together again in memory, that there will be solace and pleasure there, not just loss."

https://people.com/celebrity/keanu-reeves-i-want-to-get-married/

29

My Son I Couldn't Keep

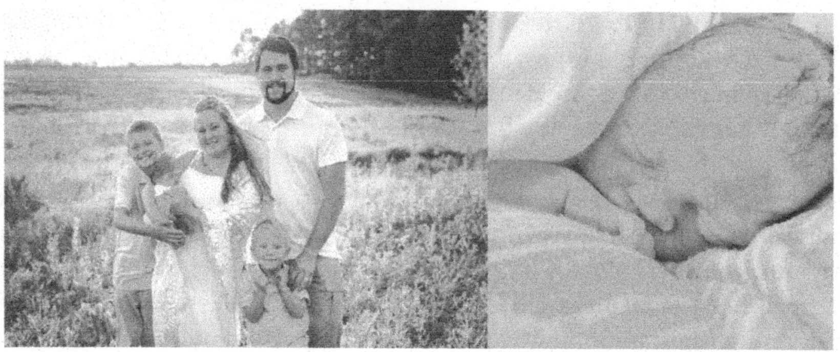

by Laura Ebel

January 21st, 2020 was, and will forever be, the worst day of my life. It all started when I woke up at 4:02 A.M. to what I thought was a painful, Braxton Hicks contraction. I went to the bathroom and everything seemed normal down below so I tried to lie back down, but it seemed as though my belly was stuck in a full-blown contraction. I sat up and instantly knew he was gone. I woke my husband up and told him that something was wrong and to get ready to go to the E.R. I went and grabbed my fetal Doppler in hopes of finding my baby boy's heartbeat, but after 10 minutes or so, I couldn't. The drive to the E.R. was excruciating; I remember telling my husband that our son was dead and he needed to prepare for just that.

We arrived at the E.R. and I was taken straight to maternity. The nurse had the fetal monitor on my belly where I could clearly only hear my heartbeat. They were stalling, waiting for the on-call OBGYN to arrive. He came in with an ultrasound machine and as soon as I saw my boy on the screen, I saw his still heart. Then came the words you never want to hear, "I'm sorry. There's no heartbeat." My response was hysteria, disbelief, screaming, "This isn't real!" But it was about to get more real.

The doctor then said, "It looks like you have suffered a complete silent placental abruption and your life is now at risk." I didn't really hear any of that; I only heard that my son was gone and I was going to have to deliver a baby that would not cry. I'd never even heard of a placental abruption before, but it took my son's life and almost took mine. The hospital was not equipped to save my life if I were to bleed out after delivery so I had to take an ambulance, 30 minutes away, to Aurora Medical Center in Green Bay, Wisconsin. At this point, I was in full-blown labor and strapped down to a bed where I wasn't able to adjust to the pain of the contractions. It felt like I was being tortured.

When I got to my room, the OBGYN came in and checked me; I was dilated to 4 cm. and fully effaced. I demanded an epidural because I felt it was unfair to go through all the pain for absolutely nothing! The doctor tried popping my water, without my permission, because he was trying to hurry things up. Because of my two previous labors, I knew that if my water broke, my baby boy would be born in just minutes. I hadn't had the epidural yet so I screamed and punched the doctor in the face.

I got the epidural. Ten minutes and two pushes later, my beautiful, still, and silent Lennix Gregory was born at 12:55 p.m., weighing four pounds, fourteen ounces and measuring nineteen inches long. He was perfect. I just cried and held him. The doctor was able to stop my bleeding; though at that moment, I just wanted to go with my son. The hardest part came three days later when I had to leave the hospital with just a little box. Life has never been the same for our family. Everyone else has moved on, but we are still heartbroken and missing our baby boy for life.

Public Figures Share Their Personal Experiences To Help Others

Annie Lennox – *Stillborn. Unknown/Undisclosed*

> "It had an immense impact on me. It made me realize that the human condition is immensely fragile and strong at the same time." "Curiously enough, I identified with those people [who suffered devastating loss from an earthquake in Turkey that occurred at the same time she lost her son] because I saw that loss is all around me… When I hear about other people's tragedies and losses, I so empathise with them.
>
> "I don't know if the pain has to come first and then you have to be in pain before you write something of any value. But it's almost like you're a potter and that's the clay you use."

https://www.telegraph.co.uk/news/celebritynews/1944539/Annie-Lennox-Sons-death-changed-my-life.html

30

Losing Anna

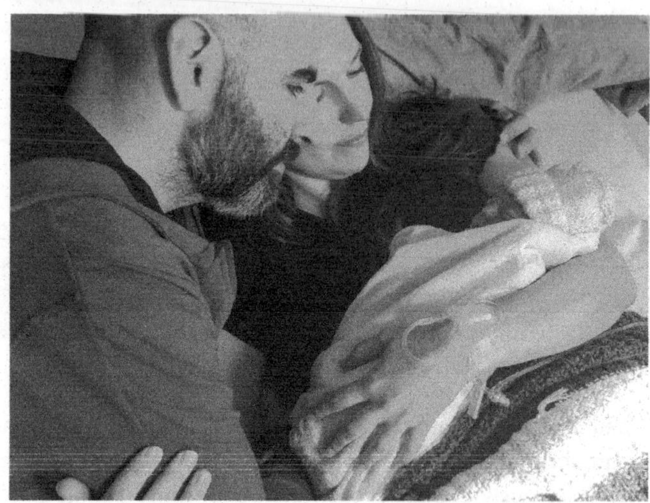

by Sarah Khouri

I'll never forget the day I lost my sweet Anna. I was thirty-five weeks pregnant and we had just finished eating dinner on our deck; the sun shone extra bright that day. I remember thinking I hadn't felt her kick in a while, so I asked my husband to put our son to bed so that I could lie down and try to get her moving. I had always been able to find her heartbeat with my home Doppler but this time was different. I couldn't find anything and I couldn't get her to kick, so I decided to go to the hospital while my husband stayed behind with our son. Looking back, I should never have gone to the hospital alone. I never thought I would be told that my daughter was gone. As I was driving to the hospital, I was thinking, *I'm over-reacting. She was kicking this morning.... Worst-case scenario, they will do a C-section and take her out early.*

Once I arrived, the midwife couldn't find a heartbeat but she told me the machine was not reliable and not to worry too much. After many minutes of searching and still no heartbeat, they took me down for an ultrasound as I was texting my husband to get to the hospital ASAP.

The ultrasound was mental torture. No one was saying anything and I was too scared to ask questions because I knew deep down that I didn't want to know the answers. I didn't want it to be real. When we got upstairs, my husband had arrived and the doctor confirmed that our daughter had passed away. We had so many questions but mostly we were in disbelief. It had been an absolutely perfect pregnancy. How could she just pass away so suddenly? It didn't make sense. The next morning, May 24, 2018, I was induced and delivered our sweet baby girl, weighing 5lbs 6oz. We named her Anna. We held her and kissed her and took lots of pictures. It wasn't enough. It could never be enough.

Her cause of death then became obvious; the cord had wrapped very tightly around her ankle. Saying goodbye and leaving the hospital without her was devastating. I didn't know how I would make it through. I had gone from having what felt like a perfect life, a wonderful husband, a healthy and happy three-year-old son, and my soon-to-be daughter. Now I suddenly felt like I had a different life and didn't know who I would be in this new, dark world. It truly felt like it was all just a bad dream and I wanted so badly to wake up from it.

I didn't think I could survive the heartache, but over time, I have come to feel like I am myself again. Maybe it's a new version of myself, but I am proud of who I am today, proud of myself for choosing to live and seek out all of the goodness that is still left in this world. A friend recently asked if I still think about my daughter. I told her I think about Anna multiple times, every single day. I can't imagine that ever changing, nor would I want it to. She is my daughter, she always will be. The only thing worse than losing her would be trying to forget her.

Early on, after losing her, I decided that if I saw a random heart shape, it would be Anna's way of saying, "Hi," to me. It was my way of staying connected to her. I'm not sure why I chose hearts but I'm so glad I did. They show up in the most random places, even my food! Maybe it sounds silly, but it has helped me so much.

Of course, there have been many other things that have helped me through the darkest days. I took several months off of work after losing Anna and my husband took six weeks off so that we could process everything together. We were fortunate that our community had a therapist who specialized in bereavement and pregnancy loss. I also found support online. Grief can be very isolating but the support groups on Facebook and Reddit allowed me to connect with other women who had suffered a stillbirth and it really helped me to not feel so alone. Perhaps the most significant step forward for me was the result of attending a weekend retreat with a small group of women who had experienced pregnancy loss in that past year. We cried together and laughed together and ultimately found strength and inspiration in each other. I left that weekend feeling a renewed sense of hope, particularly with regard to how I could honor Anna's life and spread love in her name. One of the women had mentioned a Cuddle Cot, a special cooling cot that allows families of stillbirth to spend extra time with their babies. I had never heard of it and wished I'd had one available to me. My husband and I put together a GoFundMe campaign and we were able to raise enough money to purchase Cuddle Cots for two separate hospitals in memory of Anna.

I also learned about the Wave of Light. Every year, on October 15, babies lost in pregnancy and early infancy are remembered. Monuments and landmarks around the world are illuminated in pink, blue, or purple from seven to eight P.M. to create a continuous "wave of light" throughout time zones around the world. Many cities have gatherings with music, poetry, and candle lightings. My mom and I are proud to have taken on this initiative in our town; it's a way for us to help other families shine light through the darkness while we continue to honor the memory of our Baby Anna. It means so much to us to be able to hear our baby's name read out loud. The Wave of Light has taught us that we are not alone in our grief. It is evident how meaningful it is for families to be able to honor the memory of their baby year after year through this event.

One of the biggest lessons I've learned throughout all of this heartache is to be compassionate towards myself. Some days are still very hard but there are lots of good days, too. On the hardest days, I remind myself how far I've come and I seek out self-care in the form of whatever feels good that day: booking a massage, trying a new recipe, taking a nap, reading, writing in my journal, getting outside. I've experienced many waves of grief over the past two years, some of them lasting longer than others. But over time, I've learned how to ride the waves instead of trying to swim against them.

I love Einstein's quote, "Life is like riding a bicycle. To keep your balance you must keep moving." There is no quick fix when it comes to grief. The healing process is not linear; you just have to keep going and eventually it will get easier. When in doubt, remember what Christopher Robin said to Pooh, "Promise me you'll always remember: You're braver than you believe, and stronger than you seem, and smarter than you think."

31

Reclaiming Your Indentity After Stillbirth

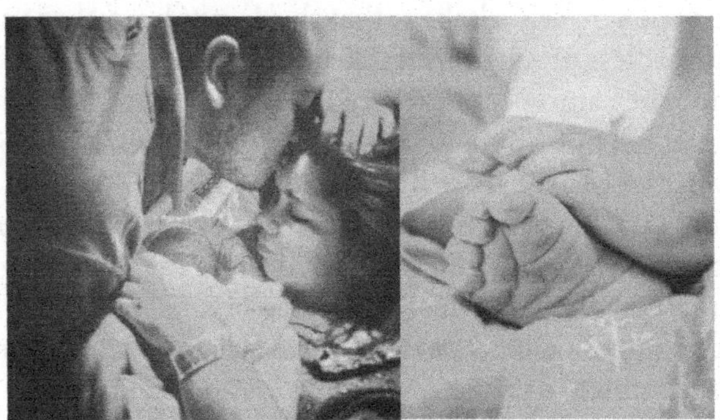

by Jessica Tamez

I lost my daughter in October of 2019. I was a day shy of 36 weeks. I had an emergency Caesarean section after showing up to the Labor and Delivery unit (L&D) early in the morning with decreased movement. They determined that my daughter was in fetal distress; I needed an emergency C-section because they needed to get her out right away. They said they were worried about her but they'd take care of her and she'd be okay.

I woke up expecting to meet my first child, only to be told that she had passed away. My daughter's dad and I left that hospital with empty arms. We left without a piece of ourselves. That sort of thing changes a person irrevocably. I have had people tell me, either out of sadness or admonishment, that I'm not the same person anymore, and they're probably right.

I definitely don't feel like I'm the same. But why would anyone expect me to be? I have definitely struggled since the death of my daughter. In some ways, I've had to figure out how to live all over again. The lines between postpartum depression and mourning my child became blurred. I stayed glued to my bed where I felt safe. Mats formed in my hair and I lost weight. I quit my job, let all my plants die, and wished that I could die, too. I felt almost infatuated with death and longed to join my daughter.

I still have days where living with the reality of my situation is difficult, when I cry because I see someone else's baby, when I miss my daughter extra and wish that I could hold her, to the point where my arms hurt. But I got better at coping, probably as a way to survive what felt like intolerable anguish. I have had days when I stayed alive because it was what others wanted.

I decided to live for my daughter's dad, because I couldn't imagine putting him through that after losing our daughter, and for my mother because I know the pain of holding your pale, cold child and wishing that you could do something, anything, to fix it. I decided to stay for my daughter as well, in an abstract way, because she would've been hurt if she knew that I had harmed myself. I believe that she'd want her father and me to be okay, and regardless of religious implications, I choose to be okay for her.

I am not the same person; there is no moving on completely from a loss this painful, but I have decided to go on for her. It's a choice that I make daily because there are still days that feel like the day that she died. I will never be the same person again, and that's okay. I have decided to embrace the truth that I'm not the same anymore. I miss my daughter and it hurts. I hurt all the time and that changes a person. I feel this way because I love my daughter, which is nothing to be ashamed of. It's something in which to take immense pride.

I hope that in reading this collection of testimonies, you can take something from my story and make the decision to take pride in your child's memory and the loving bond that you feel. Embrace yourself, wherever you are in your journey of healing. We are strong and we are not alone.

Touched by an Angel

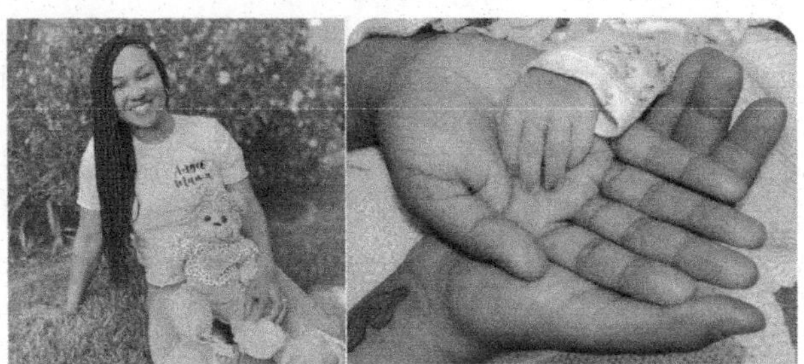

by Trinity Brown

I was waiting to meet my precious baby girl who was due on November 9, 2017. I was filled with joy and excitement. I was also nervous and filled with anxiety, not knowing what to expect during labor and delivery. Of course, everyone's story is different, and I had heard them all! I knew I would have a story to tell one day, too.

As my due date came closer, baby Noel and I were showered with so much love from family, friends, and co-workers. It seemed like the time was moving so quickly with making sure bags were packed for the hospital and ensuring that Noel's nursery was fully functional.

Everything was going so well, besides being a little uncomfortable as Noel continued to grow. On Friday, October 13, 2017 I woke up in the morning and no longer felt Noel moving. I went into the hospital, had several ultrasounds, and received the most devastating news. The doctor looked at me with sadness in her eyes and the room went silent when she said, "I am sorry there's no heartbeat." I was induced later that day and gave birth to a stillborn, Noel Alexandria. Noel was a beautiful baby girl, stillborn on Saturday, October 14, 2017 at 1:42 A.M., weighing 5lbs. 8oz, 19.5 inches long at 36 weeks gestation.

I knew I would have a story, but I didn't think it would be this story. Of course, I had heard of stories like this but didn't think it would be my reality. Every day was a challenge from that day forward. Within hours after delivery, I had to decide whether to bury or cremate my baby, ensure I had the finances to pay for the funeral services, find emotional support, and so much more. During that time, I researched and found very few resources. In some cases, there was nothing for families in Kern County, California that provided support specifically for families who have been affected by pregnancy and infant loss.

I found myself baking and cooking new recipes to keep myself busy; this became a coping mechanism to manage my grief and depression. However, that was not enough for me. I wanted to connect with others who had experienced the same tragedy. As time went by, I felt alone, and I didn't want anyone to forget my baby. I wanted individuals to acknowledge her. I needed a safe place. I had to do something not just for myself but for the community of angel parents. I decided to start a nonprofit organization.

The Noel Alexandria Foundation (N.A.F.) was founded in the summer of 2018 in honor of my daughter. The process of establishing the nonprofit was healing for me. Knowing that I was helping others gave me hope and I knew I had a purpose. I was no longer a victim, but a survivor. Now, I know that we are not alone and there is a community of angel parents to help us get through this life without our angel babies.

> *"The Lord is close to the brokenhearted and saves those who are crushed in spirit."*
>
> – Psalm 34:18

33

Losing My Daughter

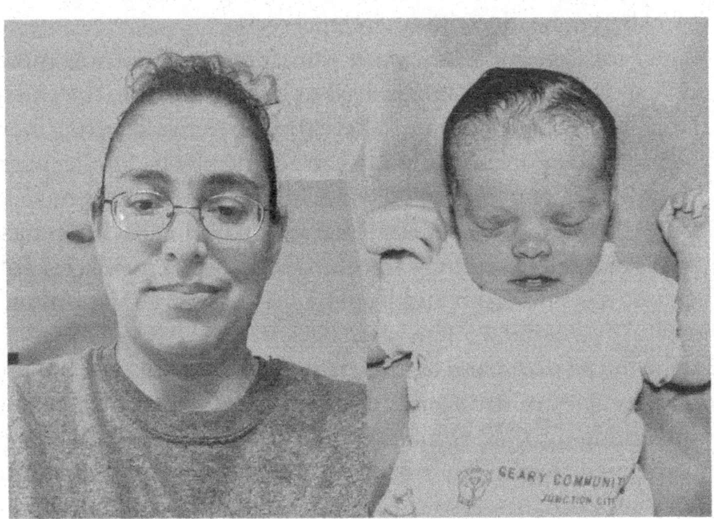

by Janel Neff

As my rainbow baby, Callista, turned twenty this year, I can't help but think about how her life and mine would have been different if her older sister, Ashlea, had lived. The pain and loss are still fresh in my mind like it happened yesterday. I don't honestly think you ever get over the death of a loved one. Instead, you find the will and strength to live on without them. My daughters are precisely one year and six days apart, to the day. It is precisely twenty-one years and nine days since the day I gave birth to my daughter, Ashlea, who was stillborn. I think about her every day. *What would she look like now if she had survived? Who would she be more like, her father or me? What kind of personality would she have? What would her likes and interests have been? What kind of relationship would she have had with her siblings?* I can honestly say, the day I lost my daughter was the worst day of my life. I would never wish that terrible fate on anyone, not even my worst enemy. Because of my loss, I learned how genuinely precious life is, and that you should never take it for granted.

It was Saturday, August 22, 1999; I was thirty-eight weeks pregnant with my second child, a little girl. I put my son to bed and I lay down for the evening with this uneasy feeling. I silently wondered, *could tonight be the night we get to meet our precious baby girl?* After a few hours, I got out of bed because I couldn't sleep. That uneasy feeling was back, but this time it was scaring me. I didn't feel her moving and my back started hurting unbearably. I called my husband, who wasn't with me. At the time, we were going through a separation. Since it was the middle of the night, I stayed in my room. Our son was asleep in his bed; I didn't want to wake him. My husband told me not to worry and try to relax. He thought it was only Braxton Hicks, not real labor. He wanted me to give it a few hours; then, if I didn't feel better, head to the emergency room.

I waited for two hours; the back pain continued and was more constant, so I called my mother-in-law. I asked her to take us to the emergency room. I told her, "I think it is time to have the baby." I woke up my four-year-old son and got him dressed to go to the emergency room. I explained to him, "It's time for your sister to be born, I think." I got to the hospital and explained to the nurse, "I think I'm in labor; I'm having back contractions." The nurse asked, "How far along are you?" I told her, "I'm 38 weeks along."

They put me in a room and hooked me up to a fetal monitor. I put on a hospital gown and a nurse came back in and checked to see if I was dilated. She did an exam, and told me that I hadn't dilated yet, but my contractions were getting stronger and faster. The doctor-on-call came into the room. Suddenly, the baby's heart rate started steadily dropping. The doctor explained to me, "Your baby is in distress; we will have to do an emergency cesarean." I was so worried about my baby girl.

An anesthesiologist came into the room and explained to me, "I'm going to give you an epidural injection in your spine. You will feel a pinch, then numbness, and you will start to fall asleep. When you wake up, your surgery will be over, and you will be in recovery. Do you have any questions?" I shook my head no that I understood. I felt the pinch, then numbness, and finally started to feel drowsy. I heard the doctor talking to the nurse and the surgeon. I could not understand what they were saying as they faded into the background, and I fell asleep.

I woke up in recovery, feeling disoriented, and groggy. A nurse came into the room and asked me, "How are you feeling? Any pain? Any discomfort?"

I told her, "My stomach hurts, and I feel nauseated."

She told me that was normal. I needed to rest a little bit longer before I could go back to my room.

I asked her, "When can I see my baby? I want to feed her."

She said, "The doctor has to talk to you first."

I fell back asleep as she left the room. I woke up again, and the nurse walked in, "Are you ready to go back to your room, Mrs. Thomas?" She asked me.

I replied, "Yes, I am. I want to see my baby; I want to feed her."

Her response was, "The doctor has to examine you first."

She took me back to my room; I asked again, "Where is my baby? I want to feed her."

"You must wait until you see the doctor, Mrs. Thomas," she replied.

I drifted back to sleep, and woke up to Dr. Khoury walking into my room.

He asked me, "How are you feeling? Any pain? Any discomfort, Janel?"

I told him, "My stomach hurts; it hurts to move."

He said, "That is normal; I can give you something for pain if you want."

I said, "Yes, please," and asked him, "Where is my baby? When can I see her? I want to feed her."

He got this sad look on his face and said, "She didn't make it. We did everything we could to save her. When we cut you open, her placenta had separated completely from her, cutting off her oxygen. I tried to resuscitate your daughter for thirty minutes, but it was too late; I am so sorry, Janel." I instantly felt the sorrow and pain consume me. I started crying and could not seem to stop. All I remember is crying and crying, thinking to myself, *My body killed my baby.*

A little while later, a nurse walked in; she held my daughter wrapped in a receiving blanket. She asked me, "Do you want to hold your baby? It is part of the grieving proces." I nodded my head, yes, and she handed me my beautiful daughter. I started to cry harder as I held my cold, dead baby in my arms, thinking to myself, *I'm never going to hear her cry, see what color her eyes are, see her smile, or feel her squeeze my hand gently*. I fell asleep with my daughter in my arms, so exhausted from crying and surgery. The next few days I was in a daze. I could barely remember who came and saw me in the hospital or what was said. But I will never forget when the nurse came back that second day and told me, "It is time to say goodbye to your baby,." So I kissed her on the forehead and told her, "Mommy loves you very much," and she took my baby away. After a few more days, I was released from the hospital and sent home. I felt consumed with pain and sorrow as I went home without my precious baby girl.

Over the next few days, we made the necessary preparations and buried our daughter. As a family, holding onto each other crying, we said goodbye to our baby girl. No parent should ever have to bury their child. To live without her is a heartache that will never heal. But through it all, we became stronger as a couple and as a family. We found strength in one another through our loss. Our failing marriage survived this loss through mourning together. Exactly one year later, God blessed us with our rainbow baby girl.

Later, I learned I had lost my baby, Ashlea to placental abruption. I will always miss my precious angel, Ashlea Michele Thomas. I am comforted a little, knowing she is in heaven watching over us.

34

Goodbye Before Hello

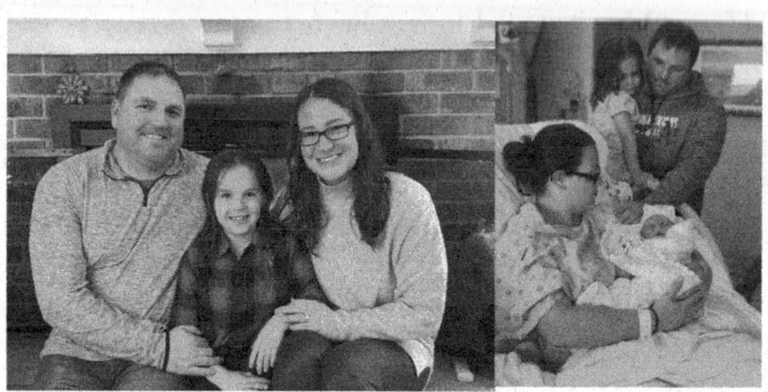

by Melissa Ziegler

I delivered my second daughter, Lillian James Ziegler, stillborn at 38 weeks on May 29, 2018. I had a normal pregnancy, only complicated by a minimal heart issue with her (tricuspid insufficiency) that we were going to have to follow up on once she was born. We were ready to welcome our new little girl into our family. Her nursery was all ready to go. Clothes were washed and put in her drawers, last minute items ordered and delivered (thanks to Amazon Prime), then our world came crashing down and was changed forever.

The night of Memorial Day, I went to bed in preparation for waking up early and going to work the next day. I woke up around one A.M., my usual bathroom break wake-up time. I got up, went to the bathroom, and had a little snack (remember, I was 38 thirty-eight weeks pregnant; don't judge my midnight snacks!). As I got back into bed and settled in, I began thinking that I hadn't really felt her move very much that night, or the previous day either. I grabbed my phone and started Googling all the ways to induce movement and what decreased movement could mean at this stage of pregnancy.

I tried all of the tips. I drank ice water to try to wake her up. I read that your stomach nerves can dull late in pregnancy as your skin stretches, so I put my hands on my tummy trying to feel any sort of movement, no matter how slight … nothing. I put my husband Jim's hand on my stomach, but he didn't feel anything either. Jim convinced me that we should go to the hospital to have everything checked out, just for our peace of mind. We called the OB triage nurse and filled her in; she agreed and urged us to go to the E.R. We woke my four-year-old daughter, Hadley, and changed her jammies because, in her four-year-old ways, she insisted on wearing a Christmas fleece top and striped purple bottoms. As we all got loaded into the car and pulled out of the driveway, I was trying to stay calm and gently explain to a very sleepy little girl where we were going and why. It had been warm the previous day, like shorts and tank-tops warm, but now, in the early A.M. hours, it was chilly. I had thrown on a pair of oversized sweatpants, a t-shirt, and a wrap-style maternity sweatshirt that had become a staple in my wardrobe in the previous months.

Jim was trying to help me and Hadley stay calm by distracting us. As we drove, he pointed out trees and asked Hadley if she knew what kind of trees they were. She said, "Lilacs, Daddy's favorite." After the short drive to the hospital, we parked in the visitor lot. It was the middle of the night but Jim pointed out how everything was very well lit because the full moon was so bright.

We checked in at the E.R., and I was then wheeled to a registration desk where they collected all of my demographic information, despite the fact that I knew it was all current and updated in anticipation of my upcoming delivery. My mind raced the whole time. Inside, I was screaming, *I DON'T CARE. HURRY UP!* I got more annoyed with each question. After what seemed like forever, I was finally wheeled up to labor and delivery.

I was put in triage room two, the same room I was in when I was in labor with Hadley. Our nurse, Melissa, helped me change into a gown and get hoisted up on the bed; my full-term body was not easily maneuverable. She started preparing the fetal monitor that I was familiar with from my days working at an OB clinic. She spread the cold gel all over my stomach. While Jim held Hadley right beside me, the nurse took the blue disc monitor and strapped it around my stomach. Silence. She tried adjusting the disc and moving it in different spots. Nothing. She asked me where they usually found the heartbeat. I told her right where it was, or really, anywhere on my stomach. They'd never had any problem finding it before. She methodically moved the disc across my stomach, back and forth, working her way up in rows. Nothing. I started to cry and held onto Jim's hand even tighter. The nurse comforted me and said, "I know this is really scary." Even with all of this taking place, I still thought our baby would be OK. Even if things were happening, she would only be a week early and would have minimal, if any, complications.

Jim left the room with Hadley to call my parents to ask them to come pick her up from the hospital and take her back to their house. We were starting to think that maybe this wouldn't be the quick visit we'd thought it would be. The nurse continued to adjust monitors and search for a heartbeat. Jim and Hadley returned and hurried into the chair right next to me. In moving the monitor, the nurse picked up my heartbeat. Hadley looked at Jim, smiled and said, "I hear it." Jim had to tell her that was mine, not the baby's.

The nurse paged my OB doctor to come to the hospital. I don't know if she was even on-call, or just came in given the impending situation. My doctor came rushing around the corner into the triage room about 3 A.M. She looked alarmed. She barely said, "Hi," and started arranging and collecting everything she would need to monitor my baby. They had to use an ultrasound machine from the E.R. because the one on that floor was out of order. The doctor seemed unfamiliar with it and frustrated that she wasn't able to use the correct machine. Based on the doctor's urgency, and repeated attempts to locate a heartbeat, Jim could tell that my parents weren't going to make it to the hospital in time to spare Hadley from witnessing what was to come.

He took her out into the hallway, and unbeknownst to me at the time, explained to her what was happening. They quickly returned while the doctor was just beginning the ultrasound, scanning for activity. I watched the monitor screen carefully, looking for any flutter, or flash, or signs of life. Nothing. No movements. No beats. Just stillness.

The doctor set the probe down on the bed next to me, grabbed my hand and looked me in the eyes. As she teared up, she said, "I don't see anything. I'm sorry." She proceeded to explain that it was too late; that there were no medical interventions or treatments to bring my baby back. She was gone. My eyes flooded with tears and I began to shake. My face started to feel hot and my ears were ringing. My mind raced trying to figure out how this could happen. *When did this happen? What am I going to do? How am I going to explain this? Why me?* I looked over at Jim and Hadley. Jim was holding it together, and Hadley sweetly looked at me, grabbed my hand, and said, "I know Mommy." I asked her what she meant. She said, "I know already; Daddy told me. I'm not going to be a big sister anymore."

I didn't know my heart could break more than it already had one minute before. *How am I going to get through this? How am I going to get Hadley through this? How can I explain to her things that I don't even understand myself?* I didn't really have enough time to process all those complex whats, whys, and hows. I had lots of decisions to make. Did I want to go home and wait to have my C-section, or have it done immediately? I barely let the doctor finish before I heard myself say, "Now."

The doctor began to explain that she thought an autopsy was a good idea. I stopped her and told her I agreed and that I was currently working at the county Medical Examiner's Office, so I was very familiar with the practices and logistics. She put her head down on the side of the bed and said, "Ah, can this get any worse?" It was then that I filled her in that my older sister, who lives in California, had just delivered her little girl nine days before. My mind flashed back to all the dreams I had of them growing up. They were going to be closest cousins even though they would be living on opposite ends of the country. They would love the same things, hit milestones at the same time…

The nurse walked in and my mind was shocked back into the moment. They started drawing blood and handing me Kleenex, making calls to reserve O.R. time and anesthesia. At some point, my parents arrived. (Looking back, it all seems kind of gray, like an old photograph). I don't remember their faces or what was said, but I remember my mom hugging me and holding me tight and both of us crying over the devastating loss. They took Hadley back to their house to let her sleep and relax until we called them to come back after the delivery.

I had to be prepped for the delivery by C-section. It was excruciating to have to go through that knowing I wouldn't hear any beautiful cries at the end. I had the spinal block and after that, Jim was allowed to come into the operating room. They had the sheet up that separated my face from my stomach and were starting to gently tie my arms out to the side when, all of a sudden, I got hot and sweaty, and it felt like someone was sitting on my chest. It was hard to breathe and I felt like I was on fire. I was freaking out. I spoke up and let them know. The anesthesiologist said he was going to give me some medicine to help me "relax." The next thing I knew, I was opening my eyes and Jim whispered, "It's over. It's all done." In that moment, I felt like Jim was talking about our baby girl's life and not the actual procedure.

I don't remember being wheeled back into my room or getting settled in there. The nurses cleaned our baby girl up and brought her to us so we could see her. I remember she seemed so big compared to how tiny Hadley was when she was born. My little baby girl was bundled up in two crocheted blankets which, I imagine, were lovingly worked on and donated for situations just like this. I remember the first thing I thought when they handed her to me was how warm she was. I thought maybe they'd had a heating pad in between the blankets. The nurses had made her a little hat with a big bow on the front. They had to use two hats to try to keep her features intact. Even when they first brought her in, the blankets and hat already showed some blood and fluid.

She looked so peaceful and perfect – almost like she really was just sleeping. I wrapped her little fingers around mine, just as I imagined she would have done. Her tiny fingernails were a purple-bluish color, a stark reminder of her condition. Her soft skin was starting to wrinkle and pull away from her tiny body.

Jim said I could name her. I'd loved the name Nola since I was pregnant with Hadley, but Jim wasn't really a fan. If I was ever going to get to use it, now would be the time. But she just didn't seem like a Nola. We had a short list of our favorite girl names. Sadly, maybe selfishly, I didn't want to use our top name. I wanted to save it for a future living child, not use it up on her. I asked Jim about Lillian – we both agreed. We hadn't talked much about middle names, and without much thought, I just said, "James." Lillian James. She was delivered at 5:10 A.M. on May 29, 2018, weighing 7 lbs., measuring 20.5 inches long. Our perfect little girl … who never got to be.

I didn't undress her or unwrap her blankets. I didn't want to see the raw and peeling skin. Her face was swollen and looked bruised from pooling blood, but my lips couldn't stop kissing her forehead. I couldn't stop looking at her, wishing she would miraculously open her eyes. I remember watching her so closely, trying to find any sign of movement. She had strands of dark hair peeking out from under her hat. I'm sure her eyes would have been dark blue, just like Hadley's, and then darkened to brown. She had cotton in her ears to try to catch any fluid that she was leaking. We had to be so careful moving her and handing her off. The blood and fluid would start to seep from her ears, mouth, and nose. I lovingly wiped her clean and was overjoyed with the chance to take care of her however I could.

Both sets of grandparents and Hadley arrived at the hospital to see Lily. They all gathered around me with Lily in my arms. I could tell they had all been crying before they even walked in the door. Hadley was just four-and-a-half and the situation was clearly difficult for her to fully grasp. Everyone got a chance to hold and talk to Lily. A photographer from the Now I Lay Me Down to Sleep organization was contacted, but she wasn't available until later in the afternoon. Given Lily's condition, that would have been too long to be able to capture her features. An OB tech, who does photography as a hobby and had worked the night before, came back to the hospital to take photographs of Lily and our family. To this day, I am eternally grateful to her. Those pictures are some of the only things we have to remember Lily. Hadley was afraid of Lily and would not hold her or go close to her. I understood; I was kind of afraid too.

I didn't yet know the calculated date of death at the time, but based on the skin slip, loss of fluid, and the shifting of her skull bones, I knew she had died before the morning I delivered her. The nurses kept telling us that we could keep her in the room with us as long as we wanted to. They gave us the option to bathe her, or re-dress her in a different outfit. I was scared. I knew from my experience at the Medical Examiner's office what was going to happen to her little body. I almost felt like I was the only one who knew what was coming. All I could think about was what I had heard said at work to parents who lose their children, "Babies go quick." They are tiny and of course don't have as much mass as adults. Therefore, the decomposition process advances much faster.

I told the nurse to come back at 10:30 A.M. to take Lily away. By then, her little face was so swollen that her profile was almost gone. She didn't look like her anymore, and I didn't want to watch her little body deteriorate any more. Her skull bones felt like they were all disconnected and floating free around her head. The fluid had fully saturated the cotton in her ears, and there was a steady stream of it running out of her nose and mouth with every minor movement of her fragile little body. The moment I knew we had to say our final goodbyes was when fluid started leaking from her eyes, making it appear like she was crying blood. I didn't want to remember her that way.

Saying goodbye was easier than I thought it would be. I didn't want to see her in that condition, so I knew we couldn't keep her. It would have been harder if her body had been in better condition. At 10:30 A.M., just five short hours after I delivered her, I said goodbye for the last time. I handed Lily over to a nurse, who took her to the refrigerated morgue so her body would be better preserved for accurate results from the autopsy.

The next three days I spent in the hospital seem like a blur. Trying to sleep, medications, sitting alone in the room with Jim, not wanting visitors, changing my mind and wanting visitors, long talks with the greatest nurses I could have asked for, trying to figure out the next steps, ordering COBRIS (certificate of birth resulting in stillbirth), contacting people and giving them the news, etc. ... until the time had come to be released. I didn't want to be in the hospital anymore.

The nurses took many molds of Lily's hands and feet. I was given a large pink hat box full of items no mother ever wants. Lily's hospital bracelet (she never actually wore it. As it turns out, you don't need to verify the identity of a deceased baby). A book, *Empty Cradle, Broken Heart: Surviving the Death of Your Baby* (this was one of the items I wanted to burn in the following days), a symbolic bracelet, a little gold ring, her height and weight card, brochures about stillbirth, etc. The hat box, all the flowers I had received, and my goody bag of disposable underwear and Godzilla-sized pads were all loaded onto a cart and wheeled into the elevator, along with me in a wheelchair. The cart and I were parked near the hospital entrance to wait for Jim to go get the car. I lasted about two-and-a-half seconds by myself before I burst into tears, ugly, uncontrollable tears. A kind older woman, who was a volunteer, came over and gave me a hug. It was a nice gesture, but it didn't help at all.

Looking back on this day, I have no idea how I did it. I get more upset about it now than I did at the time. I guess your body does just go into auto-drive when it has to, in order to survive.

My amazing co-worker, Andrea, had called the local funeral home and explained the situation and exactly what I needed. All I had to do was sign some paperwork. We left the hospital, leaving my baby girl behind. We left empty-handed, with her car seat already installed in the car, with that hat box sitting in it instead of her. We drove directly to the funeral home to authorize her cremation. We walked in and met with the funeral director, signed the three forms we needed to, and then proceeded down the stairs to look at urns. Everything inside my body was screaming, *I don't want an F-ing urn!* But instead of saying that, I asked for a catalog so I could look around and have a little bit more time to decide on Lily's final resting container.

I don't remember walking into the house that day or what I did, exactly. I do know that Jim and I both had unwavering support from friends and family. Flowers arrived for days, meals were provided, gift cards were given so we could focus on everything else. I can say for certain those days would have been a lot more difficult if it weren't for every single person who sent us their condolences, offered help, sent flowers or food, cleaned our house (mom), and thought of our family after this devastating loss.

We got Lily's autopsy report back; it was determined that her death was caused by an umbilical vein thrombosis, fetal end (blood clot in the umbilical vein). Before I delivered her, they drew about 32 tubes of my blood to test for anything and everything imaginable. Despite forming a blood clot, I do not have any clotting disorders, blood issues, or any other reason this would have happened. There is no known reason the blood clot formed (which terrifies me for the future in the event I am able to have another pregnancy).

What helped for me, in the aftermath of Lily's death, was people acknowledging our loss of Lily, not the loss of a pregnancy or loss of an idea, but the loss of my baby – who was less than one week away from being here, alive. I also really appreciated honesty from everyone. It started with the nurses who walked into my hospital room and immediately asked permission for a hug and gave condolences similar to, "I'm so sorry Lily died," or, "It breaks my heart that your baby died." I didn't want to hear soft cliché terms like "passed" or calling Lily's death my "situation." I appreciated them saying it like it was, my baby was dead, not born sleeping, (trust me, she didn't look like she was sleeping), or any other cleaned-up version of the truth.

People mean well, they really do, but they will say some horrible things in an effort, in their mind, to make you feel better. It won't. You will feel worse. And, depending on the mood you are in that day, you will react in different ways. Is it a stranger you never have to see again? Is it a family member you will interact with regularly? Are you just exhausted on that particular day? All of those things will affect your response. Whatever your response is, it is the right one. Whatever you feel you must do to be true to yourself and your child, do that. Some people aren't worth wasting your breath on. Some truly care and are just ill-informed or awkward in the face of such a tragedy. Being honest is never a bad idea. Saying something like, "I know you meant well, but what you said really upset me, and here's why.... When you say I can have other children, that makes me feel like you are minimizing my dead child's life. It is just like having two living children; having another one doesn't make you forget about the one who never drew a breath."

I've learned to be really raw and honest about the whole thing. I don't like the sappy quotes about wings and being in a better place. It's not real. That's not what happened. I didn't watch my baby grow wings and flutter off to the clouds in peace. I watched her body decompose, expelling fluids from her mouth, ears, nose, and eyes. I watched my own flesh and blood wither away in front of my eyes, with slip skin and shifting skull bones. There was no peace. There was no beauty in seeing my child that way.

The one thing that I have only recently begun to connect with is the simple truth that because I know deep despair, real grief, living hell, etc., I now know true joy. I don't sweat the small stuff. Things that used to drive me crazy at work and push me to the edge. I just drop and forget about because in the big scheme of things, it doesn't matter. If I die tonight, I don't want to have spent two hours today worrying about something so trivial and minuscule. Happy times truly are happier, because if I can get a smile on my face and laugh, while at the same time being in pain and broken, it is true happiness and enjoyment. This is not despite Lily's death, but because of it. Because of her, I have learned that I don't have to choose happy or sad; they can coexist. I can miss Lily and grieve her while still enjoying my older daughter and her delight. I don't have to pick just one. I pick both, all the time, at the same time. There will always be a missing part of me, but I feel like that forces the other pieces of me to try to shine even brighter and stronger.

The Light in the Dark

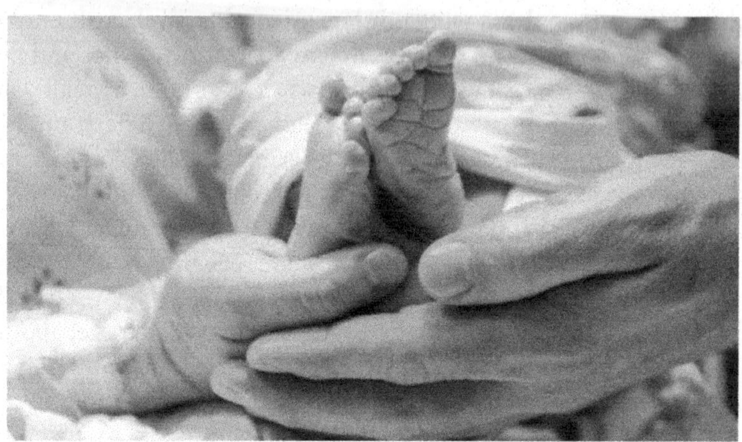

by Dustie Euler

Decomposition

I recently gave birth to my sweet son, Elliott. As I held him, I thought of all the things a newborn can be: loud, sleepy, wide-eyed and alert, healthy and beautiful. These are lovely and true descriptions for most babies immediately following birth, but not for mine. He was beautiful to be sure, but he wasn't loud. In fact, he never made a sound. The cries that were heard in the labor and delivery room were my own as I begged him to cry, too. His eyes didn't gaze into mine as I lovingly looked at him because they never had the chance to open. His eyes remained dry as my husband and I wiped tears from ours. He wasn't alert, but as his body rested on top of mine, he wasn't asleep either. He was stillborn. That's the polite way to describe what happened. That term fails to soften the harsh truth of reality, though. The fact is, he was dead and the fear of every parent is what I have been forced to face. I had no choice but to somehow discover the strength I needed to give birth to a baby I knew I wouldn't be taking home; a baby who wouldn't draw a single breath or depend on nourishment from his mother. Death altered what should have been a joyful experience and turned it into a heartbreaking one.

Blood dripped from my baby's nose, no matter how many times I gently wiped it away, and his lips were a deep cherry red because blood was pooling beneath them. His skin was peeling and I was informed by a truly kind-hearted nurse that his skin appeared that way because he was decomposing. Yes, decomposing. Let that word settle into your mind for a moment. Now, imagine a nurse telling you that's what is happening to your child. I was on the receiving end of this conversation. My precious baby, DECOMPOSING. It doesn't matter how gently that word is spoken because the meaning of it remains sharp and unable to be blunted by a soft tone of voice. Upon hearing it, I was unsettled and disturbed, to put it mildly. It's a revolting word. It's absolutely vile. Try saying it out loud as you look at the face of your child and see if you don't also shudder. (Excuse me while I go take another pill to quell the oncoming panic attack.)

Parents shouldn't have to be warned about what to expect when they see their newborn for the first time. Then again, most newborns have beating hearts. But when you're living a nightmare, the sweet nurse must delicately explain what's happening. She had to inform me that death had changed my son's appearance, so I wouldn't be startled. It wasn't his appearance that startled me, though. It was that disgusting word. I heard her, I understood her, and then I ignored her because even as his skin slipped, I still viewed him as beautiful, precious, and perfect, and it made me sick to hear her assign that word to him. He's my sweet boy, my darling Elliott, my treasured son. I couldn't bear to hear words that implied death being spoken of my child. Who can?

I collapsed when I heard the phrase, "I can't find his heartbeat. I think he's passed." I almost vomited when the doctor said, "We can't find a reason for his demise." I had to stifle my urge to scream when the midwife explained that "He appeared to have been deceased for a couple of days."

I hate those conversations and I sob breathlessly as I recall them. I hold tightly to the belief that children shouldn't be at the center of conversations involving death and thankfully, most aren't. But mine was. I can still hear those words being replayed in my mind and they absolutely break me. They make me ill even as I write about them. Those discussions have ensured my constant torment and I wrestle with them daily; I try to silence them, to no avail. Who deserves this? Who should be forced to endure so much trauma? How can anyone prepare for such heartache? Do wounded mothers ever recover from this? This wasn't supposed to happen. We shouldn't have been talking about the decomposition of my newborn. How did this happen? Babies belong in the arms of their parents, not the cold grip of death. I wish none of this had happened. I should be sitting here reading to my son, not writing about the tragedy that has consumed my life and taken his.

Facts are facts, though, and I lack the power to change them. They force me to accept the very things that have bound me to my grief: my son doesn't have a heartbeat. There isn't a reason to explain why my sweet boy is deceased. My baby had begun decomposing before he was even born and even as I held him, his tiny body was wasting away. As I choke on those bitter truths and sink even deeper into the anguish they have caused, I am also aware of these truths: his heart may have stopped beating, but my love for him grows with every beat of mine. I will always treasure and adore him because he was perfect and he will forever remain that way in my mind and in my heart. The love I have for my son has definitely changed me, but so has the horror I've experienced. That horror has thrust me into the center of suffering and it's here that I find the company of Job, another parent whose heart was crippled after terrible loss. He had great pain accompanied by even greater hope and it's his proclamation of unwavering faith in God that has strengthened mine. Job 15:13, "Though he slay me, I will hope in him." And I will too.

HEADSTONES

Grief has taught me lessons I never hoped to learn; it forced me to experience new things I never had an interest in and make decisions I never thought I'd make. Here I am, though, making new discoveries each day through the lens of grief and uncovering all of the horrific details, of which I used to be blissfully unaware. I've learned that headstones come in many varieties. I knew they were made of marble, but I assumed the material that would make up my child's headboard in future days would come from wood, not stone. He won't be resting his head in a warm bedroom, beneath a pretty white headboard with a sign on the wall above it that has a clever saying or a cute poem. He will lie in a cold grave under a marble monument with his name and the name of his twin on it, accompanied by the dates of their deaths. Their daddy and I picked the layout: the cross with the beautiful flowers on it and the lovely bible verse that will be on the back of it. I wanted to pick out which onesie and matching pair of shoes I was going to dress my son in that day, but the tragedy I was faced with required a lesson in creating epitaphs instead of newborn outfits.

Did you know that you can add vases to the side of the headstone you choose? Did you know they come in a variety of colors and it will take a minimum of three months to be completed and then placed? Did you know that when making these kinds of decisions all you want to do is scream, throw yourself over the sample monument, and sob in front of the salesman? Are you aware that you may have to stagger back to the car in a daze, hoping your nervous stomach doesn't cause you to throw up, leaving your mom and spouse to complete the process of ordering a permanent reminder that your child is gone while you empty another box of tissues? I didn't know that. I never wanted to know that. Yet, here I am with all of this newfound knowledge, just waiting for the day my children's headstone will arrive. I'll be sure to take a picture and post it to my social media accounts for everyone to see.

I'm sorry in advance for littering the newsfeeds of others that are full of happy pictures of pregnancy and birth announcements, baby bumps, gender reveals, children's birthday parties, and first day of school pictures. I, too, wish my posts were full of happy pictures instead of articles about bereaved mothers and personal stories of tragic loss. I wish I could share a picture of my son sleeping in a crib instead of a casket, but this all-consuming grief has taught me that life isn't fair, and headstones dedicated to babies are the proof. I've discovered something else about grief, though: while it resides within me, I haven't been abandoned to it. I am not alone with it. Even though it makes me feel isolated, I am not. Psalm 34:18, "The Lord is near the brokenhearted and saves the crushed in spirit." As grief continues to draw close to me, I know Jesus is drawing even closer.

Maternity leave

As I type this, I am four weeks postpartum and on maternity leave – without a baby. I thought I would be spending my days peering over the railing of a crib to see if my baby was asleep, but most days I find myself in a cemetery, staring down at his grave and straightening the flowers that were left there. I expected to have sleepless nights after giving birth, but I didn't expect them to be caused by nightmares that constantly haunt me after such traumatic loss. When I close my eyes, I want to picture my baby being brought to me from the hospital nursery, but instead I see him being taken away in a bassinet with a blanket over him, going to the hospital morgue.

I had been planning for the arrival of our first baby, but my plans were quickly derailed and I spent my time in the hospital making funeral arrangements with my family. Cremation or burial? Lillies, or roses? Should he be buried in the outfit we planned on taking him home in? No one should have to make these decisions for their child. Not ever. I bought multiple packages of baby wipes because I didn't realize that what I would really need was an endless supply of tissues to wipe my eyes. Our mailbox is full, but not with cards to congratulate us on our new arrival. Instead, we receive sympathy cards and gift cards for meals. The gift cards are welcome, not because we have a newborn to care for and are too exhausted to cook, but because grief takes far too much energy and if the meal wasn't readily available, we wouldn't even bother to eat. Who has an appetite anyway? I was supposed to be taking daily photos to capture my rapidly changing baby, but I spend hours a day looking at the few we took at the hospital before letting our baby go. I carefully study every detail of his sweet features to ensure I never forget them.

We weren't going to allow visitors after the baby was born because we didn't want to risk exposing him to Covid-19. It made me anxious to think I would have to navigate new motherhood alone. Now, I'm anxious to be left alone with my grief. I anticipated soothing a crying baby, not having to be soothed as I cried for my lost child. I used to dream about seeing my son for the first time, but I suddenly met the cruel reality that meeting him also meant saying, "Goodbye." I stayed up all night in the hospital listening to the cries of babies, but there wasn't a baby in my room. The cries that filled the halls tormented me, along with the lullaby that played with every baby born. Did they play one for my baby or did it stay silent because he was silent? I sat in a wheelchair, head down, as I waited for my husband to bring the car around to the front of the hospital and pick me up. I had to wait an extra-long time, though, because he had to take out the car seat we installed and hide it away from my view.

Our house is full of baby gear, but it's untouched. My husband frantically crammed it into the nursery upon returning home from the hospital and shut the door so I wouldn't be forced to see it as I walked from room to room. However, I find myself wandering into the nursery every day. Not to rock my precious Elliott, but to curl up on his floor and cry until my tears have dried up.

I had joined pregnancy and first-time mom support groups on Facebook, but left them to join a stillborn and infant loss support group instead. I'm surrounded by family and friends, I receive messages and phone calls, but I feel more isolated and alone than I ever have. I have been blindsided, traumatized, shaken to the core and more acquainted with grief than I ever wanted to be. The longing I feel for my son has created a deep ache that won't subside. I am convinced that there is no greater loss than that of a child. Life has changed. My priorities have changed. I have changed. Everything has changed, except God. He is the same yesterday, today, and forever, and through this, I am learning that He is still good. He is still faithful. My circumstances may have changed from what I had hoped they would be, but His character is constant. He is the Rock on which I stand.

What I Didn't Know

Nobody told me my babies would die. I've heard of miscarriage, stillbirth, and SIDS, but nobody mentioned that any one of those things was going to happen to me. And yet, two of them did. I didn't know that just two hours after being released from the hospital I would go to a cemetery to pick out my baby's burial plot. How many other new moms, who are two days postpartum, have to do that? I didn't expect to have a panic attack from seeing a pregnant woman or baby. Ads for diapers, prenatal vitamins, and onesies make me cry because I no longer have a need for them. You know what I do need? Meds to cope with PTSD. Who knew pregnancy, birth announcements, and gender-reveals on social media could trigger horrifying flashbacks? Not one person prepared me for the emotional pain of phantom kicks, my milk coming in without a baby to feed, or the silence that fills my house. I hate the silence. My baby should be crying, but I cry instead because he never will.

I was unaware that baby gifts are only a blessing when your baby actually makes it home with you, but an absolute curse when your baby dies before he gets to use them. Time now stands still in my son's nursery because everything is unused and untouched. His clothes, books, toys, and crib haunt me. There are outfits he'll never wear, stories I'll never get to read to him, and a shape sorter he'll never play with. It all sits in his room tormenting me. I had no idea that I would still feel the need to finish buying what we hadn't yet got for our son. I know he doesn't need anything, but I still needed to get it for him. Buying him additional things after he died, and knowing he won't get to use them, just added to my pain. Why did I do that? I don't suppose you know. Neither do I.

Moms talk about maternal instincts being turned on at the moment of birth, but they don't realize it applies to the mother of a dead baby too. No heartbeat? Doesn't matter. I still tried to keep my baby warm even though he inevitably became colder and colder. I wanted his hat to stay on and I insisted he stay covered with a blanket. It didn't make sense logically, but my instincts demanded it. I am now a very light sleeper because my brain was instantly hardwired to respond to baby cries at two in the morning. I wake up constantly to check on someone who isn't there. My arms physically ache to hold my baby and I have the intense desire to nurture the son I never brought home. I worry that Elliott will be scared when it storms, be afraid of the dark, or feel cold when winter comes. I'm always tempted to take an umbrella and hold it over his grave when it rains and I feel the need to cover it with a blanket when it's cold. I've contemplated putting lights around his headstone to act as a nightlight. I know all of this is illogical, but I worry about it nonetheless. I equate my maternal instincts to torture. What suffering can compare to this?

Rarely do you hear anyone mention birth, babies, and burials all in one breath, but the birth and burial of my baby took place all in one week. I watched as Elliott's casket was carried from the hearse. I tried to maintain my composure as I read a tribute to him that I had written in the hospital. I saw his casket lowered into the ground and sobbed because he belonged in my arms and not the grave. It was a soul-crushing and life-altering experience that I will carry with me until I'm buried next to my son.

I didn't plan on needing to join a stillbirth and infant-loss support group after my baby was born. I see pictures of dead babies all day long and honestly, those are the only baby pictures I can handle. When you lose your baby, you suddenly have trouble looking at living ones. I've unfollowed everyone I know who has an infant or posts pictures of an infant they're related to. I know that sounds awful, but so is death; be thankful if you don't understand.

I wasn't informed that if my husband and I went to visit our baby's grave at three in the morning, the officer patrolling the cemetery would check to be sure we weren't vandals. It might seem strange to you to visit a cemetery in the middle of the night, but when you want to be close to your child it suddenly feels very normal. It's a little awkward telling the officer that you are visiting your son while tears stream down your face, though. At least he was kind and understanding and left us to mourn in peace. Nobody warned me that I would suddenly feel isolated, rejected, and like an outcast. Yes, I gave birth, but I don't belong with the other new moms who have babies to nurse, doctor appointments to go to, and diapers to change. I just don't fit in. I'm up all night too, but it's from the nightmares and not the baby. I wish I could relate to them but they certainly don't want to relate to me. They complain because their baby is fussy and I grieve because mine is dead. They hate leaving their baby with a sitter and I hate leaving mine in the cemetery. Some are desperate for a few moments alone but I would give anything for a few moments with Elliott. I hope they know just how good they have it. It's so easy to envy them and so hard to keep the bitterness at bay. I wasn't prepared to fight those feelings off every day, but in an effort to keep them from infecting my heart, I have to persevere. Do you know how exhausting it is to guard your heart while it's overcome with grief? It never dawned on me that I would be treated as if I was contagious. I want to shout, *"Your child won't die if you talk to me!"* But that's the attitude of some women. It's hurtful to be ignored when your heart aches the most. *I promise I'm not bad luck. Please don't be afraid of me.*

There was so much I was totally unprepared for, so much that blindsided me and knocked me off my feet. I had no warnings, no clues, and no crystal ball to see that my future would hold so much pain. But the one thing I did know in advance was this: "It is the Lord your God who goes with you. He will not leave you or forsake you." Deuteronomy 31:6. I believed that verse before Easter Sunday, when my son was still alive, and I am even more sure of it now, while my heart is broken and my world is left in ruins. The truth of that verse was echoed recently when I heard a pastor say, "It is not the absence of problems but the presence of God that sustains us." And to that, I confidently say, "Amen."

36

Through the Eyes of the Father

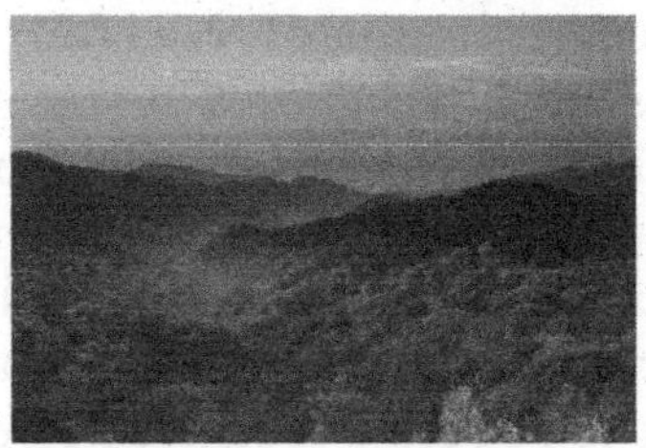

by Ed Hamilton

We had been married in June of 1966. My wife was working as a secretary and I was going to college. In the summer of 1968 we decided we wanted to start our family. I had gotten my associates' degree and was also working in the summers. I had just gotten accepted to a university in the mountains of the state where we lived. We had already found an apartment and had it rented so we could move in when school started. Sometimes, my wife would come and pick me up at work on the weekends. One day, she had a surprise for me: in July of 1968, she told me she was pregnant. That was fantastic and we were so happy.

She began seeing a local OBGYN; she really liked and trusted him. (Once I finished school and we moved back home, he would deliver our three children.) She continued to see him until we moved.

During the summer, we liked to go to a particular state park; it was a mountain range. And sometimes, we would go swimming at the pool there. On one particular day, she was wearing a blue bikini. I took a picture of her and we still have it. She was beautiful and she was carrying our baby. Today, it means so much to look back to when we were so excited and happy.

The summer moved on and we were finally living in the mountains. Right across the street was a hamburger chain and we both worked there for some time. As time went on, both of us got jobs at the university. She was working on several projects for the university until she landed a job as a secretary. I got into a Work Study program. Some of the professors could not drive and my job was to drive them to off-campus lecture classes and then back to the school. While they lectured I could study.

After about two to three weeks, we decided to go home for the weekend. It was a two-hour drive. We had a Ford station wagon and I dropped the seatbacks down so my wife could stretch out and rest; I didn't want to disturb her or the baby. On the way home, I had the radio on with the Beatles playing

"Hey Jude." We continued to go home as much as we could. At Christmas, my wife was wearing a purple vest and purple skirt and a white blouse. Her mother took a picture of her; she was so beautiful and radiant and so pregnant. After Christmas, we stopped coming home but our family came up to visit us.

One night, we were in bed and my wife said, "Give me your hand." I did and she placed it on her stomach. I could feel the baby just a kicking her stomach. That was one of the greatest moments in my life. We both laughed and I said, "If it's a boy, he might be a football player." Oh how special that moment was for us. She felt the baby many times but for me, in the future, that moment would become extremely important. That was the one time I got to come in contact with our baby. That was a little human being just waiting to be born and come into our world and our life.

We moved into another apartment after the first of the year, which was great for us because we lived next to some people from home. My wife had someone to visit and talk to when I was working. Friends and cousins and neighbors threw her a baby shower. A crib, basinet, chest of drawers, toys, and clothes were all in our den/living room. They were there waiting for our baby. We were so excited and happy.

I remember taking her to her doctor when I wasn't working at the school. When I was working, she had our car and drove herself to his office. The doctor said everything was fine with the baby and my wife was also doing well.

One night, we were in bed and one of the slats the bed was on slipped, and the bed fell. There we were, on the floor, just a laughing. We got up, put the slat back where it should have been and went to sleep.

In January, she quit working. It was hard being in the apartment by herself but she had our friends next door. She still went to the grocery store with me and we would go to the movies on the weekends. The movie theater was cheaper on the weekends because the college students would go home then, so the theater showed lesser-rated movies. We were glad to see anything. At that time, we were also attending the First United Methodist Church and had a great minister.

In one of my classes, we had a project to do about anything we wanted, as long as it pertained to health. I was doing mine on infants and the cause of infant deaths. Our state had a high rate of infant mortality. (Even today, the death rate for children is still too high.) One reason was that some women were not able to afford prenatal care because they didn't have any insurance. At that time, I don't remember health insurance; if there was any, we didn't have it. I remember studying about President John Kennedy and Jackie's children that had died at birth. My professor, who was a woman, told me one day she couldn't understand why I was writing my report on infants until she saw my pregnant wife with me at the grocery store.

In early March, we began counting the weeks until she would deliver. On the 20th of March, when I came in from being off campus, my wife said, "I think the baby is getting ready to be born." The next morning we were waiting for the doctor at his office. When he arrived, he took my wife right on back to check her. He told her, "Everything is going fine, you can go on out to the hospital." He told her the baby would be born about 9 p.m. that night, March 21, 1969. We got to the hospital and the nurse took my wife to her room.

My wife wanted me to go on to class, saying I didn't need to be sitting around the hospital since the baby wouldn't be born until later that night. I did not want to go but I did and it was one of the worst mistakes I have ever made. I still think about it to this day. I should have stayed. I did not learn until later that my wife was breech and my mother was breech. The doctor had not mentioned anything to her about a breech birth. I do not know if there is any significance to that and the baby's birth or not. I also found out doctors don't know everything about babies and their arrival time.

At about eleven o'clock, I couldn't stand the tension anymore and cut my next class. I went by the apartment on the way out to the hospital. I called the hospital to see how my wife was doing. The nurse that answered said the doctor wanted to speak to me. He came on the phone and said the baby was a boy. *So far, nothing to worry about, everything was normal; we had a son!* In his next breath, he shattered our world forever. "The baby was breech and the cord was around his neck." I was holding on to the wall at that point; I really don't know why I didn't pass out. That was it; I can't remember, "I am sorry for your loss," or anything. The doctor was gone when I arrived at the hospital and I didn't see him until the day he checked my wife out.

On the way out to the hospital, my religious beliefs were tested. I had a talk with God I would not normally have. I asked him, "How can you be a loving, kind, and merciful God and let this happen to us?" I had grown up in the Baptist church and my wife was a Lutheran and now we were attending a Methodist church. We had attended church faithfully our whole lives. What had we done to deserve this? My wife was the most compassionate, loving, and kind person you would ever want to meet. Not one person from the church came to visit us, not even the minister. We talked to him later and he said he was not aware of the death of our baby. I do believe him.

When I got to the hospital, the nurse took me to my wife's room and naturally, she was crying. What she told me was another story about the doctor and the nurses. She had received a saddle block. You don't do that with a breech birth; the mother can't push. They had to call the doctor and tell him the baby was on the way and would be born without him if he didn't get out there. My wife said he was there when the baby was born. The idea behind him being there earlier when the baby was breech, is that he could have done a cesarean section. We had friends whose children were born successfully via C-section. Once our son was born, my wife frantically asked, "Why is he not crying? Why is he not crying?" I don't have any idea who had to break the news to her that he had died.

I had called our parents when I was in the apartment and they arrived at the hospital. My father-in-law and brother-in-law took our baby back to a local funeral home. He would be buried on Saturday, March 22, 1969. My father-in-law took me out to the funeral home. We went in and I got to see my son. There he was, fully developed, a big baby boy. He was perfect in every way. In hindsight, he looked like our other three children would look when they were born. (They all looked like their mother and so did he.) There are some things they didn't do then that I think they do today. The parents get to hold the baby. That helps with closure. No, it doesn't stop the pain and suffering, but you can get by that part by holding and loving your baby; just holding them in your arms.

The next day, I went with my mother and my next-door neighbor to the baby's funeral. I saw our baby in a coffin. He was in a blue outfit someone had given to us at the baby shower. I regret someone didn't take a picture of him. Everyone left the funeral home and went out to the cemetery for the graveside service. The minister who did the service was from the Baptist church I had attended. I thought he did a good job; the scripture he read was very appropriate. Friends of the family, neighbors and uncles and aunts and grandparents were there along with my mother and my father-in-law and brother-in-law. I can't remember much that was said to me that day, but my uncle told me, "You are young and you can have more children." That was coming from a man who, along with my aunt, had lost twins. When my uncle passed away about 20 years ago, I told my aunt that I had never forgotten what he told me that day at the cemetery.

Buying a cemetery plot is not usually what two twenty-three-year-olds do in the first years of marriage. This is not what I had envisioned when my wife got pregnant. Life can be cruel and sometimes it plays favorites. Later, we bought a plot in a better part of the cemetery and our son rests there today. We still go out and put flowers on his grave. There is something about a cemetery that can be soothing.

We left the funeral and went back up the mountain. Since my wife had been in no shape mentally or physically to attend the funeral (she had carried a very big baby), I went out to the hospital to be with her. That night, some friends from home came up to visit her.

The next day, before the hospital released my wife, the doctor came in to see us. I would be lying if I said I wanted to meet with him. He told us that he wanted to deliver another child for us. The rest of what he said I can't, and don't want to remember. My thoughts were, *You had your chance and if you had been here when you should have been, we would be taking our baby home. You could have done a C-section and been a hero to us.*

My wife still had to go out to his office for follow-up visits. Other things happened with her that I don't want to write about; they are still very private. It is ironic that doing my student teaching I had our doctor's son in my class. I treated him no different from anyone else. He was someone's son, like all the other boys in my class. All I wanted to do was get off that mountain. (We did not go back for ten years. We took our children up there to see where we used to live, and out by the hospital.)

When we got to our apartment, my mother and my wife's mother were there. All the gifts were in plain sight. Later, they were taken apart and put in a closet. We went to our bedroom and closed the door and we cried until we couldn't cry anymore. I think it was more like the wailing that is mentioned in the Bible. That was not the last time we cried for him. We have cried just about every year on his birthday. There is no way to describe how we felt. Only people that experience the loss of a child can feel that kind of pain: The feeling of being a total failure, dejection, and that life has dealt you its most devastating blow. It was made worse by friends and cousins having babies when we had lost ours. I was happy for them but I'd just as soon not hear about it. My mother-in-law stayed for a week or so with us. I don't want to discuss how my wife's life went after my mother-in-law left.

We did not have anything to fall back on. Some couples have other children and they can gain strength by loving them. We had each other, but a woman that has lost a baby needs something extra to love and to get love from in return. I would have never thought an animal would have done the trick for my wife. While I was writing this, she asked, "Did you write about Tweet-Tweet and how he saved my life?"

My in-laws had brought us a parakeet; my wife named him Tweet-Tweet. She told me stories of how she would be in the bathtub and he would be running along the side of the tub and just jump in. She would be brushing her teeth and he would be on her toothbrush while she was brushing and he would be pecking on her face saying, " I love you, I love you." He served a great purpose for my wife, holding her together until we had another baby. The smallest things can make the biggest difference sometimes.

On the day she reminded me of the parakeet, I told her I sometimes had a vision of the doctor who delivered our three living children and whom she was seeing when she first got pregnant. In this vision, he delivered our first baby in the hospital at home and he had done a C-section and was lifting the baby out and removing the cord from around his neck. Sometimes you have to escape reality for just a minute or two.

The summer after we lost the baby, I was working at the First United Methodist church. After I got out of class in the mornings, I would go over and take the children that the church kept during the day for working parents out to play. We played games of all kinds, softball and things of that nature. When I arrived, all the children would be waiting for me up on the mezzanine, near the banister. I can still see the face of one little guy. I will remember him as long as I live. His name was Bart and he had Downs Syndrome. He was always happy and loved to play.

My wife would usually walk over to the church after she got off from work. Sometimes, we took some of the children home; they did not have a ride and were picked up in the morning and taken home in the afternoon. One Friday, Bart's mother said they were going on vacation the next week. That afternoon, his mother and Bart laid down to take a nap. Bart never woke up. I felt so sorry for her; they'd had him for about nine years and then he was gone. Life can be cruel for us all.

In March of 1970, I had graduated and was back home teaching and coaching. In April of that year, we were blessed with the birth of a son. After what had happened the first time, I did not want to go in the delivery room. I remember when the doctor came out (the same doctor she was seeing when she first got pregnant before we moved to the mountains in '68); we were in the elevator and he told me everything went fine. I asked, "Well, what do we have?" and he said, "A boy."

I called my mother—no answer. I called my wife's parents—no answer. Well, I had to tell somebody so I decided to go to their homes to tell them. When I got outside; I saw they were walking into the hospital. I hugged my mother and said, "It is a boy!" After some time, I was finally allowed to go in my wife's room while she was nursing. I got to see my son! He looked just like her, and just like his brother in heaven.

We went on to have two more wonderful children, daughters that we love and cherish so much. It's been fifty-one years since we lost our first baby boy but we have never stopped loving him.

In 1998, my wife and I were in bed when the phone rang. I answered; it was our son. He said, "We are going to have a baby and it's going to be a boy!" I handed the phone to my wife. "What happened to dad?" he asked and she said, "He is crying." Yes, I was crying; it was a cry of joy and happiness, not sadness. He wanted to know if it would be okay to name him after our first son, his brother whom we had lost at birth. I felt like a ton of bricks had been lifted off my heart. It helped so much.

My wife and I drove to Florida when our grandson was born. We also went to his baptism. We now have one more grandson and three granddaughters. We feel so lucky to have five healthy grandchildren. When my youngest daughter had given birth to her first daughter, her doctor told her to consider herself lucky to have a healthy and normal child. She said there are so many things that can go wrong during their development.

Everyone who experiences the death of a child feels loneliness and helplessness. One thing that gave me strength and hope was from a book a friend of mine wrote. At the beginning of each chapter was a message or a bible verse. The one I remember said death can never win because love is as strong as death and death can never take away the love you have for someone. It can't take away the good memories and the good times. I can still feel our first baby boy just a kicking his mother's tummy. That memory can never be taken away from us. Yes, we still hold each other and have a cry on his birthday but I will never be ashamed to cry for him because of all the love he brought us.

In the summer of 1968, after we knew my wife was pregnant, she and I were trying out a new 2+2 Mustang. While we were driving, the Ohio Express came on the radio singing, "Yummy, yummy, yummy, I got love in my tummy." We had love in her tummy. Every time we hear that song, it takes us back to a time of happiness and joy because we were going to have a baby.

Rest in peace, DGE.

37

You Will Never Have a Cloudless Sky, But the Sun Will Shine Again

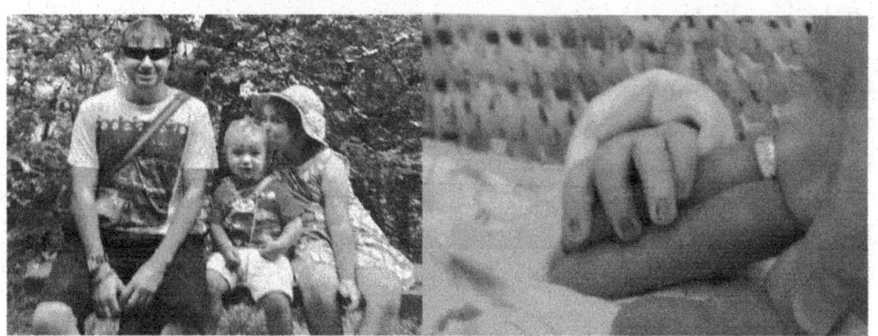

by Daniel Harding

My wife and I were very happy that we were pregnant. Leighton was our first together, as I have a daughter from another partner. The pregnancy seemed to be going well, but my wife did experience a sharp stabbing pain in her lower back and side, and her blood pressure was high. The midwife was happy, as there seemed nothing to worry about. Leighton was growing very well; he had long legs that we could see from the scans. He was always moving and kicking. We were in bed one night and Leighton kicked so hard he kicked me in the back!

Leighton seemed to hide from the midwife when she was using the Doppler. We went to see her for the 39-weeks check-up. On the Tuesday, his heartbeat was fine with no signs of what was about to happen to him.

The weekend came and Saturday was good, no problems. Sunday came. My daughter lives with us and the three of us decided to go out for the day. We went to Torquay. We stopped for lunch and my wife said, "He's quiet today; I've not felt him move." I said he might be resting. I bought my wife an ice cream to see if that would make Leighton move. He didn't move at all.

My wife and I decided to go to Accident and Emergency (A&E) at Exeter Hospital as we lived in Exeter at the time. Unfortunately, my daughter had to go through it with us the whole time. We went straight to the early pregnancy unit, which is shut on weekends; eight rooms full of equipment not being used. The doctor tried to find a heartbeat. At first, we were both laughing because, as I said before, Leighton liked to move about and try to hide. I looked at the scanning monitor and the doctor turned it away from me. Then the laughing stopped and I looked straight at my wife. There was horror on my face as I looked at her. The doctor said, "I'm so sorry; I can't find your baby's heartbeat."

My world came tumbling down on me. What started out to be a lovely day turned into my worst nightmare. I'd seen things like this on TV and thought, *Wow, how do you get through that pain?* I was truly broken; I couldn't help save my son or help my wife with this pain.

The next step was to remove my son. The doctor had to put a tablet into my wife's womb to start labor. I phoned my mother-in-law and told her the bad news. She said they would come and get my daughter so she could stay with them. They live in Plymouth. The first thing my father-in-law did was hug me, even though he's never been a hugger.

They sent us home but we had to come back Monday morning. My wife and I were devastated and lost. We got home and just sat on the sofa, no TV on or anything. I felt helpless and a failure. We went to bed and my wife woke up screaming and crying, "I want my baby! I want my baby!" How do you comfort your wife when you're broken? I cried with her and held her until she stopped, but she did it twice more that night.

We got up in the morning to go to Exeter Hospital for my wife to give birth to our son naturally. We were taken to a nice room but it was near the labor ward so, now and again, we could here babies cry. The good thing was that the sun was out and it was going to be a beautiful day.

The consultant came in and explained what would be happening: it would be a normal birth, as if our son was alive. He also said we would have to arrange a funeral for Leighton; as his was a full body, the hospital wouldn't get involved with that part. Fair enough. That wouldn't be until the post-mortem was done and Leighton was given to our chosen funeral directors. We also met our midwives; one was a student.

The hospital fed me and gave me a mattress to sleep on. For me, there was unlimited milk for tea and coffees, just to try and keep my mind busy. I had a book but I wasn't in the mood to read. TV (with quite a lot of channels) and phone calls were also included. But again, we had no interest in anything. We just kept in contact with our family.

Nothing happened on day one of trying to give birth. We all couldn't believe it; this was a nightmare but it was very real and cruel. I was angry with God; I said horrible things to him. *Why take my son and not me? What has Leighton done that I haven't?* My wife kept waking up in the night, screaming, "I want my baby!" That was the hardest part. I just comforted her; that's all I could do – that, and cry. I'm supposed to be the man who protects my family. I couldn't even do that, or help my son.

In the early hours of the morning, my wife went into labor. She requested the epidural, which the doctor put in. The midwives were very nice and totally understanding. Leighton wasn't born until the afternoon of July 13, 2013. I cut the cord. He was cleaned and weighed, then passed to my wife. We both broke down in tears. So did the midwife, who has been doing this job for many years.

Leighton was so beautiful. He had very long legs; when I held him, his legs were past my elbow. He looked so peaceful. We took photos to make it feel normal. The midwife took his hand and foot prints and made a card for us; that special touch made me feel humble. The midwife said we could go home with Leighton if we wanted to. Some parents have done that. We didn't; we stayed all together. The midwife brought in a cooling block to go under the travel cot. It was a very hot day, so we put him in that for a bit and he also had to go in the cooler for a bit. That was the worst: not seeing Leighton; I wanted to cuddle him all the time. I never wanted to put him down. *He's mine and no one should take him from me now*. My wife had a catheter put in due to the epidural. She had blood taken and the after-birth was sent away for testing. It was horrible. The next day, I asked the midwife if she would arrange for Leighton to be blessed in the chapel by the minister, which she did. She put a blanket over the basket so no one would see Leighton as I carried him through the hospital.

Our own midwife came to see us and Leighton. She was in tears, too. It wasn't her fault. She left. Then the consultant came in to explain the next steps, which were to send us home in a day or two, have a post-mortem on Leighton and register his death.

Leighton was sent to Bristol, as there were only two doctors that were specialists in child post-mortems. We had another day at the hospital with Leighton, in and out of the cool room because of the heat. We spent a total of four days in hospital. The midwives told us that the post-mortem would take four to six weeks. The consultant and the midwives were very good to us. Then, we had to go home. We left Leighton behind in hospital and came home empty handed, which was very, very hard. Our midwife gave my wife injections to take each day for two weeks and we scheduled follow-up appointments.

We were both a mess and at a loss about what to do. The doctor signed me off work; he was totally understanding. I couldn't show that I cared. I was broken and hurt. I needed time to heal. To keep my mind busy, I bought Leighton a couple of paper airplanes and dinosaurs, which I decorated with yellow tissue paper and varnished, so he'd have some toys with him.

I worked in a nursing home at the time as a care assistant. The manager was very understanding. Time passed so slowly. My daughter came back from my in-laws when the school year started. My wife was offered six sessions of counseling, but none for me. My wife said, "No. Not unless my husband can come as well." They said okay and we had one together but my wife went to the rest alone.

The counseling sessions were held at Exeter Hospital, right below the labor ward where we lost Leighton. It was painful and cruel. The last time we had been to the hospital, we left our baby there. As we went in, we saw a pregnant woman smoking. We saw new babies going home. We just sat in the corridor crying.

Three weeks later, we were hit by another bombshell. The midwives were wrong. The post-mortem would take sixteen weeks, not four to six weeks as we were told.

On the weekends, we went to the in-laws' house and helped tidy the garden just to keep busy. I had no interest in anything. I wanted to swap with my son. *Take me instead!*

My wife and I had to register Leighton's death at the registrar's office. We were told that we would not have to wait in the same waiting area as the other parents with their newborns. That wasn't the case. We sat and waited. I was angry and very upset. The lady called us as if she had not made us wait at all; no apology, nothing. I didn't want to eat. It was our first wedding anniversary and we didn't want to celebrate that.

Dark times were ahead with no let-up of the pain and grief. I got in contact with Marget, the minister who wed my wife and I, and asked if she would do the service for us. She said to come and see her at her house; we had a cup of tea with her. She was very understanding as my wife and I were both were in tears. We had a long chat as to what music we should have. We chose a song from the Russell Crowe film, *Gladiator*. We can't watch the movie or listen to it anymore. I will never forget it. To this day, we have never been back to Torquay.

Weeks passed … I was still off work and my wife was meant to be on maternity leave. We chose a funeral director in Plymouth and met with her. Her name was Leighanne Wright. We bought Leighton some clothes and she dressed him in them. She said she would be in touch when Leighton was ready. We felt Leighton shouldn't be alone in Exeter so we chose to have him cremated in Plymouth. I'm not from Exeter and neither is my wife so we decided it would be best if he was with family in the remembrance garden in Plymouth. The funeral director advised us there probably wouldn't be any ashes, as Leighton was small. We chose a yellow teddy bear. We used to call him our yellow baby.

We finally got a phone call from the funeral director to let us know Leighton was there and that we would have a chance to see him one last time. My wife didn't want to but I did. I had an hour with him in my arms. I will never forget that moment in my life, ever. I cried so much. The hour went so quickly; it wasn't fair. The day came to say our last goodbye to Leighton: the 8th of August, 2013. My family from Hastings came down for support, as did our friends. I bought a yellow tie. I say it's Leighton's tie; I wear it on special days. The only thing I wish I had done differently at his funeral was carry him. I regret not doing that very much. To this day, it hurts.

I've never seen a counselor about the loss of my son, but we have done other things to help us cope. We always celebrate Leighton's birthday. If it falls on a weekend, the whole family goes out; if not, then it's just the two of us. My wife made a box for Leighton's pictures, his armbands from the hospital, and his blanket. We put his name on the box: Leighton Benjamin Harding. It's a yellow box. All the cards from the family are in there too, as are Leighton's foot and hand prints. And my wife and I have both agreed that Leighton will go with the first one of us that dies. I'm a Freemason and my lodge donated some money to the hospitals in Devon and Exeter. The funeral director that dressed Leighton, Leighanne Wright, also lost a baby. She set up "Little Things"; she makes clothes for premature babies and babies that have died.

My wife and my nursing home manager both decided that I should go back to work; I felt I wasn't ready. But would any time be a good time? I went back to work. I was very low and depressed. Life for us just went on. Eventually, we decided that the time was right to have another baby. It took us a while, but we found out we were pregnant on Mother's Day. My wife and I and the whole family were over the moon, but because we lost Leighton, it was not an easy pregnancy.

We had our rainbow baby, Faith, who is nearly six now. My wife had another miscarriage at twelve weeks, but then our son, Lewis, was born; he's nearly two. Both keep us busy. But Leighton is the first thing I think about, and the last. I still miss him loads. He's still my boy.

Public Figures Share Their Personal Experiences To Help Others

Robert Munsch – *Full Term. Unknown/Undisclosed*

"I'll love you forever,
I'll like you for always,
As long as I'm living,
My baby, you'll be."
(From the book *Love You Forever*)

"I made that up after my wife and I had two babies born dead. The song was my song to my dead babies. For a long time I had it in my head and I couldn't even sing it because every time I tried to sing it I cried. It was very strange having a song in my head that I couldn't sing.

"For a long time it was just a song but one day, while telling stories at a big theatre at the University of Guelph, it occurred to me that I might be able to make a story around the song.

"Out popped Love You Forever, pretty much the way it is in the book.

"My regular publisher felt that it was not really a kid's book and I ended up doing it with another publisher.

"One day the publisher called up and said, 'This is very strange. It is selling very well in retirement communities in Arizona. It is selling in retirement communities where kids are illegal. This is supposed to be a children's book. What is going on?'

'Grownups are buying it for grownups!'

"In fact, it turned out that parents buy it for grandparents and grandparents buy it for parents and kids buy it for everybody and everybody buys it for kids.

"As a matter of fact, everybody buys it for everybody. That's why it sells a lot of copies. I think it's my best book. [...]

https://robertmunsch.com/book/love-you-forever

The Life of Emory

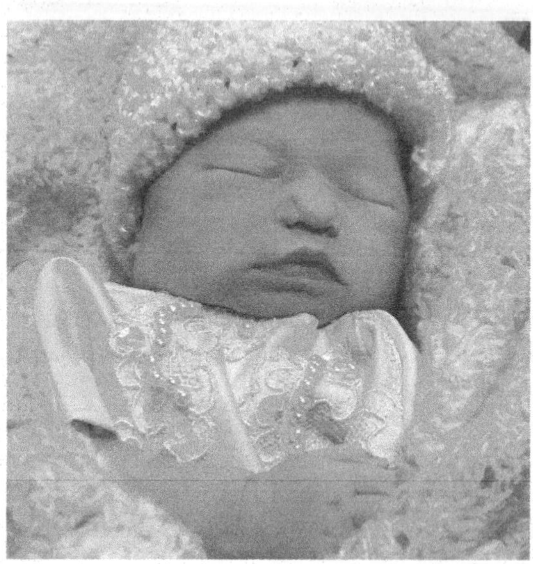

by Sunshine Penny

I have been with my partner, Reggie, since January 2016. I have two children, ages 16 & 7, from a prior relationship. He has one son, who is ten, from a prior relationship. We have very much wanted a baby together! We suffered four, first-trimester losses in the first three years of our relationship. After miscarrying the last one at home, I was done! I no longer wanted to try to make our blended family complete ... so I scheduled an appointment to get on birth control. However, before I ever made it to the appointment, I started spotting before my cycle was due.

I decided to take a test. To my surprise, it was positive! I felt scared, happy, anxious, nervous ... every emotion possible. When the spotting didn't stop, I figured I was miscarrying again. We went to the hospital and, to our surprise, the baby was fine. I had a small subchorionic hematoma. After a few days, I stopped bleeding.

The first appointment came and went. Baby was great! Strong heartbeat, perfect growth! We stayed cautious, as we didn't want to get our hopes up, again. But we were SO happy! At about twelve weeks, I was working the third shift and I started bleeding again. I was terrified! I left work early, went home, and checked her heartbeat; she was fine! The bleeding stopped less than 24 hours later ... we breathed a sigh of relief.

The first and second trimester came and went. Before we knew it, we were seeing the doctor bi-weekly. We knew we were getting close. Everything was great! I had a baby shower at work and another with family. We were so ready, so prepared to bring our baby girl home! (The baby girl Reggie had always wanted.)

Wednesday, February 5, 2020, we left the doctor's office happy. Baby was strong and had a heartbeat of 156 bpm. We were four days away from her due date so we scheduled an appointment for the following Monday to have a stress test done, if she didn't make her arrival before then!

When we went home that evening, everything was normal. There was a bad storm on Thursday, but nothing alarming for us. The kids went to school and came home. I got the kids ready for bed that night and sat down at my kitchen table. I was randomly scrolling through my newsfeed on Facebook when I came across a post made by another expecting mom. She expressed her worry for her baby's lack of movement. And at that moment, I realized I hadn't felt my baby girl move since the night before. I jumped up! I went to the bedroom, laid down, and immediately started searching for her heartbeat. I couldn't find it! Reggie jumped up and got dressed and we anxiously drove, ever so quietly, to the hospital. I pushed on my belly hoping she would move. But, nothing.

We were taken to labor and delivery. A nurse came in and searched for her heartbeat. And again, nothing! The nurse got the mobile ultrasound machine. As she put the wand on my belly and went across my baby girl's heart, there was no movement. The room was quiet. We knew. I knew! She called in the doctor ... more silence ... no movement on the screen. The doctor looked at us and said, "There's no heartbeat." Ohhh, those three dreadful words, again!

She was gone! My Babygirl was gone! The nurse started to cry as I screamed, "OH GOD! NO! ... NO! ... NO!" Reggie and I held each other and just bawled our eyes out! Reggie literally took off into the bathroom and started vomiting! I just cried ... and cried.... *How could this be? She was fine!* We were supposed to be bringing our baby home in a few days! *How could she be gone?*!

I called my mom, and Reggie called a few relatives. My mom came to the hospital. I just didn't know how I was supposed to give birth to a baby that I already knew would not be breathing. I was then admitted to start the induction process. I was given Ambien to help me sleep as my cervix ripened. But I didn't sleep; I just cried until my eyes were red and puffy!

We started Pitocin around five A.M Hours came and went.... My mom picked up my sixteen-year-old son and came to the hospital for the delivery. My seven-year-old was not allowed to come because of "flu season restrictions." That really upset me more, as she was so happy to finally have a sister; and yet, she couldn't even meet her! As I felt her crowning, Reggie called my mom and the doctor; everyone walked in the room as she was entering this world! I was 39 weeks 5 days and at 2:45 p.m. on February 7, 2020, I gave birth to my sleeping daughter, Emory Reign Ashe; due to what the doctor's say was a silent placental abruption.

She lay on the bed ever so silently. I just cried and cried and cried. She was really gone! I had prayed and hoped so much they were wrong, that by some type of miracle, she would come out crying. But she didn't. She was silent, and peaceful. And yet, at that very moment, my heart broke into a million pieces. My life changed forever!

Why would God bless us enough to carry, prepare, and anticipate this beautiful little girl's arrival for 9 months and yet, take her before we even got to see her eyes, before we ever got to hear her voice or even got to learn who she would have been. I will never understand why God cut Emory's life so short.

I still don't know how I even managed to get through each day. For the first month, I was dead inside! I didn't want to live anymore. Grief took over my entire being! And the truth of the matter is that I was put on the 7th floor. Sadly, it took that for me to understand that I still have two children that I have to raise, two children that depend on me and need me daily. So, giving up wasn't an option. I had to stop being selfish in my own grief and misery and start thinking of my living children. If it weren't for them, I can't say where I would be today.

I started seeing a therapist for a little while. It was the only place I felt I could grieve because I spent most of my time putting on a brave face for my children. I still do. I don't like them to see me sad. My seven-year-old was so protective of my heart. Every time she saw babies in the store, she would guide me down a different aisle so I wouldn't see it. I love her so much for her protection over me, but I also know that I have to be strong for her. I am supposed to be her protection, their protection! All of them! Even Emory! But I couldn't protect her life. I feel like I let her down. My body let me down, and in turn, I let Emory down! My body didn't do what it was meant to do when she needed me most! That haunts me a lot of my days.

Emory was cremated. We have dedicated an entire wall of our living room to her! Her pictures, memorial, personalized items, and her urn all sit in our living room. We have NO shame to put her in a displayed frame for the world to see. Just because we were not blessed enough to get a photo of her breathing does not mean she isn't worthy of being framed. She is a HUGE missing piece of our life, of our family. My children, along with myself, all have urn necklaces. I wear mine daily. It brings me peace. I have also dedicated my entire right arm to Emory. I have started a sleeve tattoo in her memory. Getting the tattoos done is therapeutic for me when dealing with my grief.

It wasn't until I gave birth to a stillborn child that I learned just how big the community is, just how common stillbirth is. One in one hundred women will suffer stillbirth! That is mind-blowing considering that it is hardly ever spoken of. And when it is, people get uncomfortable and change the subject. I've learned it's up to us, the ones who've suffered this tremendous heartache, to speak up and speak out! Therefore, I share Emory's life with the world, because her life means the world to me!

I Had A Son

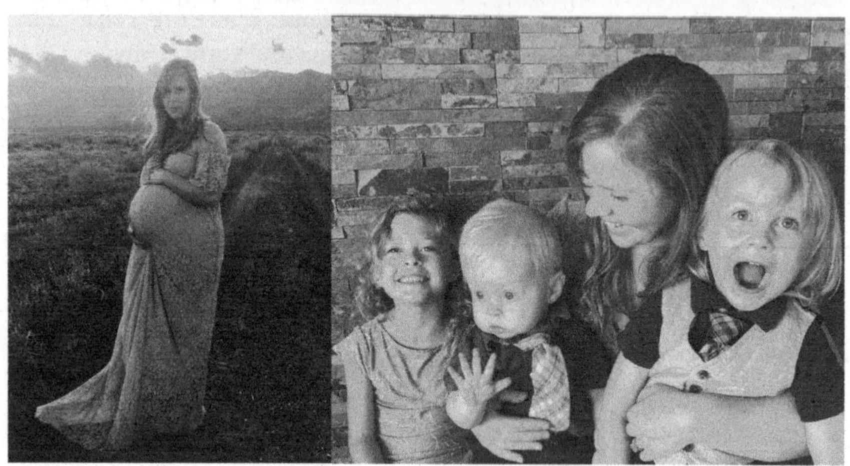

by Michelle Fulton

I had a son.

His name is Cole Vaughn Taylor Fulton.

I grew him for nine months. I knew him for nine months.

My husband, our daughter, and our living son only knew him from the few kicks and hiccups they could feel radiate from my belly. He knew us from the muffled sounds of our voices speaking or singing to him on a daily basis ... but he never got the chance to see our faces or feel us embrace him. After he was born, my husband and I held him and wept over him. But that was all we got.

Two years prior, I had forced myself to read a story written by a woman who had lost her full-term baby just before his birth. The pregnancy had been normal and the baby healthy until he unexpectedly lost his life. I had forced myself to read her story, and other such devastating articles, because I liked having knowledge on my side. I am a naturally optimistic and positive person, so it never put me into a tailspin, or paralyzed me with fear ... it was just painful information that I kept filed away. Before reading the article, I had believed stillbirths only occurred from serious health conditions in mother or baby or because of tragic cord accidents during birth. I was shocked and concerned to find out that was not the case. How I wish I had taken that cue to do more research ... but it was a sad and stressful subject so I felt that measured exposure was all I needed.

At around thirty-eight weeks pregnant with my third child (we chose to wait until our children were born to find out their sex; we liked the surprise of it – like opening a gift at Christmas), I woke up at three in the morning, panicked because I couldn't feel Baby kicking. Fearful thoughts of death crept into my mind. I usually only felt Baby move from around eight p.m. to midnight so the lack of movement shouldn't have upset me on such a deep level, but I couldn't shake my unease. The next morning, I told my mother about it. We reminisced about my similar anxiousness and fears when I was waiting for the imminent arrival of my son, Turner. So it was a normal anxiety and I decided to put it out of my mind to ease the stress I was feeling. I didn't tell my husband, Christopher, about it; he didn't need the added stress either ... and besides, it was just a silly qualm that had struck me in the middle of the night.

When scheduling my next prenatal appointment, my midwife, Tesa, asked if I wanted to see her on Monday or Friday. For no particular reason, I said Friday. Friday came and we were about to head out the door when she texted saying she wouldn't be able to make it and would the following Monday be okay? We set the time for two o'clock, Monday, and I got back to nesting.

I had never had a strong nesting urge when I was pregnant with my other two children but I made up for it this time. For weeks I had been tidying, organizing, hanging pictures that had been sitting in the closet for the last two years, wiping dust off surfaces I had never even thought about before, and doing laundry: loads and loads and loads of laundry. My mother had come down from Canada to help us prepare. We were both like whirlwinds spinning through the house, erasing every speck of dust (I wish) and returning each toy or trinket to its rightful place.

My daughter, Bella (now four), had been born prematurely at thirty-four weeks and five days and Turner (now two) had arrived at thirty-nine weeks on the dot (very quickly and unintentionally in our bathroom!) Each day that passed that I carried our baby number three was worthy of celebration. It was getting down to the wire but the house was clean, the baby clothes were folded and organized, the freezer was stockpiled with pre-made meals, and in case Baby decided to arrive at home like last time, the birth pool, hose, Chux pads, and heating blanket were at the ready, and I had made the bed with a layer of plastic between two sets of sheets. Christopher and my mother had even taken full-term maternity photos for me (they were something I had always wanted but never got with my previous two) and I felt like a beautiful, fully prepared goddess. Practically everything on the to-do list had been checked off–something I had never accomplished during my previous pregnancies. Now I was ready, and because I was ready, I was anxious for Baby to arrive.

We were receiving calls and texts constantly: *Is Baby there yet?* Anticipation was high. With his arrival about to occur any day, I pushed my fear aside. It popped back up every so often, but like most of my fears, I rationalized that the possibility was there but the probability was not high. I should have looked up the statistics; the probability was far higher than I realized. Instead, I chose to focus on the joy and elation I would feel when my beautiful baby actually made his debut and I could hug him and kiss him and hold him close.

I had just gotten over what I had believed to be sinusitis and bronchitis and was battling hormone-triggered cold sores on my face ... *Just let the cold sores clear so I can snuggle with my baby,* I thought. And miraculously, they did—in days, rather than weeks. And as I rejoiced in my health, I immediately got sick again. That, I was okay with: Baby would get all my antibodies from nursing, and a little phlegm wasn't going to keep me down when I had my infant in my arms.

All Sunday, I had the longest and strongest Braxton Hicks. I knew my body was getting ready; I couldn't have been more pleased. That night, I stayed up a little later than usual to mop the kitchen floor—maintaining cleanliness was a high priority; I knew that after Baby was born, only minimal housework would get done for a long time. After the floor was done, I sat down to relax and watch a little TV before bed. That's when Baby normally made his presence known, when I stopped moving around for the day. But that night, Baby seemed unusually inactive. Again, my fears resurfaced as I patiently waited for a kick or hiccup. Eventually, I felt him stretch and that was enough to stop me from completely losing my mind with worry. Baby's movements had become less dramatic as he grew and ran out of room, but when there was no more movement after I lay down to sleep that night, my uneasiness intensified.

Why didn't I call Tesa right away? Did I think it was too late at night? Did I just not want to be a bother? Was I so afraid that something was wrong that I was in denial? None of that should have mattered AT ALL. This was my baby's wellbeing and I, as his mother, should have let my concern drive me to get checked out. None of my petty conscious, or subconscious, reasoning should have stood for anything in the face of my baby's very life.

Early the next morning, I messaged Tesa with my concern. "Drink some cold water, eat a snack, then count kicks for an hour." I did just that. Right after eating a banana, I had the urge to go to the bathroom (there was not a lot of room for things other than Baby during that stage of pregnancy.) As I relieved myself, I believed I got a series of good kicks from Baby ... *or was it just my guts vehemently protesting?* (Not unusual for me.) I sat down and remained still for an hour. Fifty minutes in, I got a single stretch ... *or was it another Braxton Hicks?* I had been hoping for more, but something was better than nothing. I let Tesa know and tried not to stress. *That wasn't Baby's normal awake time and we would be seeing the midwife in just a few hours.* It was then that I let Christopher know I was anxious to see Tesa and why.

Christopher and I had been working on a contract for five months. At the onset, we believed it would be drawn up and signed within a few weeks. But the weeks dragged to months, until we were financially stretched past our limit and our comfort level was a distant memory. It sucked a lot of the excitement out of having our baby, but with amazing support from our family and friends, everything was going to be okay; we were afforded enough breathing room to still feel that spark of happy anticipation.

After five long months, the contract came in that day: Monday, February 10, 2020. For whatever reason, our lawyer had it for two hours before we found out. We asked him to send it to us a.s.a.p. It arrived in our inbox at one p.m. It took forty-five minutes to drive to Tesa's office. We had to print the contract, review it, sign the last page, then scan it, and send it back. We were going to be a little late, but we could get it done.

As we were about to walk out the door, the lawyer called and said we had to scan the whole contract with signatures and send it as a single PDF. So, after figuring out how to do that, I had to scan all ten pages. Luckily the printer made fast work of it, and we would still only be a little late for our appointment. After sending the new file, we got another call from the lawyer; the resolution was too low. I then adjusted the resolution too high (just the first page took three nail-biting minutes to scan) before I found a happy medium (which still took too long in my opinion). I texted Tesa to tell her I felt like I was in the seventh circle of Hell and we would be much later than expected. We rescheduled for four o'clock and when the contract was finally signed and sent, we headed to the appointment.

Once there, Tesa checked my blood pressure; everything was in order. We talked about getting a stress test. She would check Baby's heartbeat then we would head to the hospital to make sure everything else was fine. On the examining table, Tesa checked Baby's position ... good position ... but when she was feeling around, he didn't kick back, which was his normal response. As she held the Doppler to my tummy, there was no reassuring, thump-thump, thump-thump. My breath caught in my throat. Baby's heartbeat had always been very strong and Tesa had always found it immediately, even when Baby had been very small. I didn't breathe in the hopes that I could hear better. As she passed the wand over and back across my belly with no sound, tears sprung to my eyes. I looked over at Christopher with a mix of shock, fear, hope. I pleaded for sound.

"How upset should I be?" I asked Tesa, through my tears.

"Give me a minute," she responded. She pushed the wand from different angles and tried to find even the quietest beat. "It doesn't look good; you need to go to the hospital."

I leapt from the bed, now crying hysterically that we had to leave immediately. Christopher quickly conversed with Tesa as I stumbled outside in a nightmare of a daze. I was sobbing loudly as I approached the car where my mother and other children had been waiting patiently.

"What's wrong?" my mother called out the window in alarm.

"She can't find a heartbeat," I gasped. "We have to go to the hospital!" I awkwardly slid into the car and got myself buckled in as Christopher rushed into the driver's seat. He set off at break-neck speed; the nearest hospital with a labor and delivery wing was an hour away.

I prayed. I messaged my sister and my sister-in-law. They both tried to reassure me; they both urged me to try and stay calm. I envisioned the best outcome: *something was wrong with Baby. His heartbeat was so soft that the Doppler couldn't pick it up. We would get to the hospital and they would do an ultrasound. Baby's heart would be beating weakly. "We need to do an emergency C-section, now!" I would be rushed into surgery and they would save my baby. I would wake up and be reunited with my infant through tears of thankfulness.*

I posted on Facebook that my baby needed prayers; they came flooding in. Deep down I knew it was probably too late but what did I have to lose? If prayers and good vibes and positive thoughts could have any impact, then I wanted the whole world to know what I was going through and to focus their energy on my baby's survival.

We made it to the hospital in record time. Christopher dutifully lit a fire under anyone who wasn't moving fast enough to get us the help we needed. After taking an age to get behind a curtain and into a hospital gown, they came in with another Doppler to look for a heartbeat. I didn't want another Doppler; I needed the ultrasound. But they listened with the Doppler; they passed that damned wand over and back and over and back across my belly until one nurse gave up and another came to try. The endless effort was unbearable as each second passed and there was still no heartbeat. After straining with every fiber of my being to hear the faintest sound, I was relieved and terrified when they brought in the ultrasound machine.

There was Baby on the screen. I knew where his heart was; I could clearly see that it wasn't pumping.

I was immediately transported to an alternate reality because this couldn't be my story. In my story, my baby's heart was beating. He was alive, and I would get to see him soon, and our lives as a family together would flourish for so, so many years to come.

I stared at that little heart, still as stone. I felt like if I concentrated hard enough, if my will was strong enough, the electricity from my grief would leap into that heart and it would jump back to life, an unexplained miracle that I would marvel at for the rest of my life… but all the prayers, and all the concentration, the sheer will, and electrified grief didn't change the inevitable outcome: my baby was gone. The suddenness and finality of it was tortuous.

I just needed to hold him ... but he was trapped inside of me. I would have to give birth to my baby, knowing that he already had no life left in him.

Christopher and I cried and tried to speak. He went to tell my mother; she was sitting in the waiting room with Bella and Turner. While he was gone, I was taken for another ultrasound in another room. I bounced between numb silence, and hysterical sobbing that swelled from every cell in my body.

When Christopher rejoined me, he tried to transfer his strength to me. "This will bring us closer together; this will not tear us apart," he promised. He held my hand and stroked my face and spoke to me more openly and broken heartedly than he ever had before. Despite all the ups and downs through our marriage, in that moment, when I needed him the most, he was all the best parts of the man that I had married nine years earlier. I felt like if he hadn't been there, every part of me would have become disjointed and unglued and pop apart and would never fit back together again.

He stayed with me as I was taken to another room, the room where I would do the hardest thing I have ever had to do (and pray I will ever have to do) in my entire life.

Tesa arrived. Christopher had to leave to take our children and my mother home. He would come back as quickly as he could.

Through my tears, I managed to update my post on Facebook. I knew I wouldn't be able to bear the prayers and well wishes continually coming in for the health of my baby when I already knew that he was gone. I had to let everyone know; I needed them to direct their love and strength to me and my family so that we might survive what we were facing.

My cervix was effaced and dilated enough that I could be given Pitocin to induce labor. I also chose to have an epidural. My other two births had been natural and drug free; I had wanted this one to be as well, but without a living baby, the motivation for that had changed. I didn't want to feel anything.

I talked to Tesa. She held me as I cried. She helped me get to the bathroom when I needed to go. We joked in moments of numb, suspended reality. She made sure the nurses took the best care of me. She kept me together while Christopher was gone. She even brought me a box of soft Kleenex (the endless supply of hospital tissues seemed to be made of sandpaper and every time I wiped my eyes or blew my nose, it added another level of physical pain to the hellish mental anguish I was already experiencing.) She answered my questions and listened to me ramble through the mess of thoughts that clogged my mind.

What if I had just asked for a stress test when I first woke in the middle of the night in fear? Why did I choose to have my prenatal exam on Friday instead of Monday? Would it have changed anything if I we hadn't rescheduled to the following Monday? What if the contract had come in sooner? Was it because I had slept on my back? Was it because I was stressed? Was it because our pellet stove had clogged in the night and filled the house with smoke? Why didn't my body just go into labor when Baby was still alive? Was it the tuna I ate that once, or because I ate tinned baked beans? Was it? What if? Why? Why? Why? I easily got lost down that rabbit hole (for a long time after the birth too), but each heart-wrenching question led in circles to the same place: both me and my baby had been perfectly healthy for the entire pregnancy, until the tragic end. Now, my baby was gone and there was nothing I could do to bring him back, even if I had all the answers to all the questions that haunted me. Without some definitive, divine foreknowledge, I could not have changed my actions because I am who I am and I am human.

Because my son left our world before he ever entered it, I turned to every otherworldly possibility to try to find some kind of answer. But all I could find was comfort, there were no answers. And as thankful as I was for all the comfort, support, and love, none of it would bring my baby back to me ... and that was all I wanted. The only thing I could do was keep moving forward, step after step into the dark world of birthing a baby that I could not raise.

As the contractions started to intensify, I utilized the hypno-babies tools I had learned to have a natural and pain-free childbirth. It helped. It would have been glorious and exciting and empowering but now it just helped me cope; that in itself was invaluable. I had been so looking forward to the birth, but now I had the worst mix of never wanting to go through it, and needing it to happen immediately.

Christopher came back. He had become a rock and I was moored to him, trying to weather the most treacherous and tumultuous storm I had ever experienced. With him and Tesa and the nurses, I had a small community of people to hold my hand, speak lovingly to me, hold me, and listen to my heart breaking. I could not fathom going through it alone.

Every contraction was more emotionally painful than it was physically uncomfortable. The thought of getting the epidural brought me some peace but as it was administered, the awkward, strange, unexpected, and raw feeling that paralleled my spine made my cry out in frightened pain. The technician tried three times; each time, he gave me another shot of local anesthetic. All the while, I was slumped over a pillow, unable to move as each contraction intensified. After the epidural (which took over twenty minutes to administer), I had another unpleasantly strong contraction. Two more followed with lessened force; I thanked God that it was starting to work. But immediately after that, I transitioned and needed to push. The epidural had not numbed me completely and the urge, the pressure, and the trauma of it all were back in full force. The doctor wanted my knees up and my legs in stirrups. I didn't want my legs in stirrups; I wanted to twist on my side. My body knew what position I needed to be in but the nurses held me in place. I don't like to use foul language but I was cursing, and crying, and with the next contraction I screamed out "WHY?!"

I focused on my muscles doing what they should be doing, moving Baby down and out. I could feel his head; I didn't fight it. I let every muscle stay relaxed, and when I needed to push, I pushed. I told Christopher that he should leave if he needed to but he stayed by my side the entire time.

As my son was born, I was hit by a wave of relief.

Unable to see below my waist, I imagined two scenarios. The first was as it should have been: the joyous birth of a healthy baby. But the second was the horrifying nightmare of reality: the limp and lifeless body of my child sliding silently into the world. Both scenes still haunt me.

"Is it a boy or girl?" I asked.

"A boy."

I cried.

Cole Vaughn Taylor was born at 11:59 p.m. on February 10, just days before his due date.

A nurse lightly cleaned him, and swaddled him at my request, and handed him to me. As soon as he was in my arms, I feverishly unwrapped him. I thought I had wanted him bundled up but some primal part of me needed to hold him, skin to skin—as I had imagined for the last nine months.

He looked so peaceful, like a healthy, sleeping newborn. I studied his precious, perfect face. I held his hand and kissed his forehead. I rocked him in my arms and gently shushed him as if he was fussing. I couldn't help it. Oxytocin was flooding my body and bonding me to my baby that I would never take home. I willed his heart to start beating, his eyes to open. My heart jumped as I curled his hand around mine and I thought I felt resistance in his little fingers. My will was so strong that it made my mind capitulate. But my baby boy was indeed gone, and those few brief and tender moments were the only ones I would have with him. All the prayers in the world would not make him open his eyes, would not start his heart, would not bring him back to us.

I looked at him and a startling wave of anger rushed through me. I was angry at him for leaving me, for breaking my heart, for being so strong, and then not strong enough, for succumbing to whatever it was that took his life. I had cursed my body for failing him, and cursed myself, and cursed the universe, and that all felt fine. But the anger I felt towards him caught me off guard; I felt like I was burning up from the inside. I was angry at the most innocent being in the whole world. I held him close. I loved him more than anything but no matter how hard I tried, I couldn't hold him close enough to change anything.

I held him, and Christopher held him, and when we couldn't bear it any longer, Tesa held him for us. He grew cold and the color fled from his face. I knew I couldn't look at him anymore; I needed to remember him as warm and pink, right after his birth, as if he was just sleeping.

The hospital staff created a keepsake box of handprints and footprints, pictures, a lock of hair. I knew I wanted them because of the devastating articles, written by bereaved parents, that I had forced myself to read so long before. I was thankful that their tragic experience was able to guide my decisions at a crucial time when my own brain refused to function.

Before she left, the photographer asked if I would like the hat that Cole was wearing to go in the keepsake box. I said no. At the time, I didn't know why: maybe holding on to too much would make it harder to let go? Later, I regretted it; I should have kept everything I could. But in writing this, in processing, there was something about taking the hat off his head, facing the fact that he didn't need it anymore; at that time, it was just too painful to acknowledge on top of everything else.

We decided to have an autopsy done. We were warned it would probably not give us any answers but we decided that if we didn't, we would always wonder, and if there were any answers, maybe it would bring a modicum of understanding, and thus peace, to us. They took Cole out of the room and left us there to comprehend our loss.

I wanted to go home; I needed to see Bella and Turner, but even though I did not have my baby, I had given birth, and the doctor said I needed to stay in the hospital to be monitored.

Christopher spent the night with me. They made up a separate cot for him but I needed him to hold me. He climbed into my hospital bed and held me in his arms all night long. We cried and coughed and talked and cried until we passed out from exhaustion and grief. Unconsciousness was sweet oblivion but after only an hour, the nurse woke me up to check my temperature and blood pressure. There was no more sleep after that.

I was given a questionnaire to determine my level of depression. "Over the last seven days you have felt …" I made a note at the top that I would fill the form out taking into account only the last twelve hours because everything had changed so drastically in that time. After a woman evaluated my response, she said, "Your marks are fairly high on the depression scale." I wondered if she had ever lost a child, and how she felt just a few hours after finding out.

I had been told that I would be discharged that day so I could get home as soon as possible. My blood pressure had always been perfect during the pregnancy but now it was reading a little high. I had tried to talk to a friend and then my sister-in-law on the phone but all that came out was hysterical sobs. My blood pressure was high because I was upset but the doctor decided to keep me longer just to be safe.

After Christopher had to leave for the day, I felt trapped and numb and alone. Every part of me wanted to flee the stark room in that regimented hospital but instead, I was stuck there, left with only my thoughts and my questions and my sorrow. I was empty, in every sense of the word ... just empty. Nurses came and went; food came and went. The TV was on; I half listened and half watched though glazed eyes.

Anything I normally enjoyed doing, or anything that was usually a good time-killer brought me no comfort of distraction. I couldn't read, I couldn't surf the net, I couldn't write, I couldn't play a game, all I could do was sit and cry.

I did manage to converse via text with a few people. All the anticipation of getting to share the birth of a beautiful baby had nowhere to go. I wanted to tell everyone his name. I wanted to share his picture. I needed everyone to know that I'd had a lovely baby boy, but how could I do that now? He was gone. There was no joy, no pride, no wonder at the miracle of life, only complete and utter desolation. I asked our closest family members if I could share his photo with them. If they said yes, I did. It brought me a little relief.

My best friend said she wasn't sure if she should tell me, but she felt moved to. She had just found out, the same day I lost Cole, that she had lost her first pregnancy. We cried and held each other through our typed words. It was early on for her, but she and her husband had been trying for months, and this had been her first positive. Whatever the differences were between our experiences, there was a kernel of truth that we shared, a thread that joined us in the pain of a lost child; the pain was the same even though our circumstances were different. We were able to comfort each other, not only with our words and love, but by the very fact that we were not alone in what we were going through. I wish with all my heart that her text had said that she was pregnant instead of the reality of loss, but suffering her heartache with her, and her with mine, we found solace in each other and solace in knowing that our children were together.

Christopher came back in the evening. He brought a meal that had been lovingly prepared by friends, and he told me things would get better once we got home; being with the children would help. Again, we shared the hospital bed and settled in each other's arms and prayed for dreamless sleep to take us. My bronchitis-like symptoms had become progressively worse and my own coughing awoke me throughout the night. Each cough brought a shocking, stabbing pain from a pulled muscle under my right breast while I was forcefully reminded of my nonexistent bladder control (thanks to the catheter for the epidural). I couldn't breathe through my nose and when I breathed through my mouth, I coughed, and when I coughed, I wet myself and felt like I was literally being stabbed through the heart. Christopher was a saint to share the bed with me for as long as he did.

After little to no sleep, the sun rose again and I was more than anxious to return home. The wait to be discharged was long and unbearable. Nurses and social workers and who knows who else came in to speak to us. Some were cold in their lack of understanding, others were horrifyingly chipper, but most were real, and compassionate, and offered their most heartfelt sentiments to us.

Finally, we were given the green light to leave. It was all I had wanted since giving birth but when I walked down the hall and saw the exit, a force slowed me down and held me back. I couldn't leave, not without my baby. I was supposed to be leaving with my beautiful, healthy boy. My body heaved with grief as I crossed the threshold; I clung to Christopher to steady myself.

As we drove home, the desert hills glimmered yellow with the very first flowers of spring.

It was better to be home. Seeing and holding my living children started to stitch my heart back together. But being with them wasn't without difficulty. One of the first things my daughter said to me was, "Don't worry, Mommy, the new baby isn't dead." My heart jumped, despite everything that I had just been through, my first visceral reaction was one of hope. It made no sense to feel that way, but somehow, because everything else felt so surreal her words were like a lifeline that said, "See, it was all a bad dream, now you can climb back here, back to the reality you were expecting"; but of course, that wasn't the case. She went on to tell me that the baby was floating in the sky, up in heaven, and one day, we would all move to heaven to be together again. I held her tight and told her I loved her as I unsuccessfully tried to choke back my tears.

The following days and weeks were a challenging mix of appreciation and thankfulness for my living children, finding the right words to explain the situation to them, fighting to expose them to a healthy amount of tears and grief without getting lost in my pain, my changing hormone levels, and role-playing. Bella's favorite game while I was pregnant was putting a baby doll under her shirt so she could "grow her own baby." The loss of Cole did not change her enthusiasm for this same game. In fact, now she wanted me to play the expectant mother as well. Despite the pain, we played to process our feelings.

In looking at my son, Turner, I saw where Cole should have been in two years. There was a brief point in my grief where I couldn't stand to look at my surviving son for the distress it caused me. Every time I looked at him, I cried and felt like my insides were atrophied because that beautiful glimpse into the future was always poisoned by the fact that it would never come to fruition.

My milk hadn't come in, and I didn't want to go near the pump until I absolutely had to. At 6:00 A.M. on my first morning at home, I absolutely had to. A plugged duct made an irritating, hard lump so I massaged it as I pumped, alone in the dark kitchen. I had to pump multiple times that first day to manage the discomfort; the lump remained, and the milk did not drain quickly. Luckily, cold cabbage leaves in my bra took care of the lump in a matter of hours. After that, I pumped once a day, then once in two days; in between, I waited as long as I could stand it. I wanted my milk to dry up. Everything was a painful reminder: the bruise that covered my left hand from the I.V. that was attempted multiple times; the pinprick mark on my right hand, in the crook of my elbow, and halfway up my arm from the other IV attempts and blood tests; the lochia that leaked from me continually; the lack of bladder control; the inability to pick up my kids; the stabbing pain in my chest ... the sooner I could eliminate the reminders of what I had lost, the easier it would be for me to move forward and heal.

I had waited too long to pump on the last day (nine days after giving birth). I didn't know it would be the last time but as I sat on the bed, painfully engorged, and started the pump, my daughter burst into the room. I yelled at her to get out. I was too damaged, too vulnerable, too hurt. She quickly retreated and I cried out in desperate, emotional pain from the guilt of yelling at the first child I was blessed with, and the physical relief that being was provided for me by a machine instead of my newborn baby. The tears came heavy and hard, and my whole body shook as I pumped away the last of the milk that I would ever produce for Cole.

I couldn't speak on the phone. I couldn't see people. Friends and family, far and near, reached out and I couldn't face any of them, even through the computer. Tesa offered to be a go-between for those who were intent on helping us. I couldn't have been more thankful. Another very dear friend set up a fundraiser to accommodate our grieving and any unexpected costs we might face. We were overwhelmed by the support and love that was shared with us from our family, friends, community, and even people we had never met. Knowing that so many had truly loved Cole, even though he was never able to join us earth-side, touched us deeply. Many said they had no words. That spoke deeply to me because that was exactly how I felt: there were no words to express every emotion, every "what if," the guilt, the grief, and that in itself brought me comfort. Mere words fell short; anything I said seemed grossly inadequate. And so, sharing no words became an unspoken understanding of the difficulty of the situation, and that in itself brought me comfort.

Truly thoughtful gifts were sent to us: a bulk pack of Kleenex boxes, each with a different biblical passage about loss and strength handwritten on the side; Epsom salts for a soothing bath; aromatic oils to help with stress, anxiety, and grief; other self-care products; and candles that had been lit with prayer.

My brain stopped working at its normal capacity (pregnancy brain was one thing, but this was like pregnancy brain further depleted by half). I was making mistakes, forgetting things, and my forgetfulness was making life so much harder. I got overwhelmed very easily; it took me much longer to accomplish any task; I lost my ability to think and plan ahead with the detail and precision I had before; and words escaped me, not only in conversation, but also how to spell them. I had always been a strong speller, but now, it was like I was just learning. I would write things like "imotions" instead of "emotions." I would run though every possible spelling of homonyms, and I still could not remember which one was correct. It has gotten better but I still make these mistakes. I hope that with the passage of time, and as the pain and trauma become more manageable – once my capacity is not being fully engaged with processing – I will regain my former abilities.

I didn't feel enthused about anything. Having never experienced depression before, I found it frightening. There were moments of peace, and some of numbness. The rollercoaster of feelings was actually helpful in that I never stayed in one state for too long: sadness, guilt, isolation, numbness, tranquility, forgetfulness, devastation. The ride was exhausting, but I never wanted to be stuck in one emotion. I just wanted things to even out a little, smooth out the track so it was more of a kid's ride than an extreme loop-de-loop.

The first few evenings at home were strange; the numbness seemed to take over once the kids had gone to bed and we tried to relax a little before we went to sleep ourselves. I felt as if maybe the last nine months hadn't happened at all, all the sickness, the discomfort, the sacrifices.... Throughout my pregnancy with Cole (which had been the most uncomfortable by far), my motto had been: *"It will all be worth it."* And it was. I vomited joyously because I knew it meant I was growing a baby. I reveled in my surprising weight gain as I ballooned to almost 200lbs because it meant I was creating life. The exhaustion was to be celebrated because it meant most of my energy was going towards expanding our family... and all of these little discomforts were only temporary. But when I got home, and there was no new baby in my arms, it was like none of it had happened, because if it had actually happened, where was my baby? My mind grappled to make sense of it, and in those numb evenings, I just gave up trying because it was all so senseless. It made more sense to believe that none of it had happened at all.

I had loved my giant body while I was pregnant. It was a little alarming, how big I was, but it became like a game: will I hit the 200 mark this time? I knew it would be hard to work off the weight, but I had eaten healthy the entire pregnancy and kept up with low-impact exercise on almost a daily basis. I just get big when I'm pregnant; the same thing happened with my other two but it was always worth it.

After I lost Cole, I hated my body. It was big, awkward, painful, sweaty, disgusting. The awkward phase between pregnancy clothes and regular clothes wouldn't have fazed me if I'd had Cole in my arms. But now, people were asking me in the supermarket when I was due, or if I was having a boy or a girl, and all I could do was silently shake my head before I burst into tears. A couple of weeks post-partum, I started to look like I was just heavy instead of pregnant, so that was a blessing, but I still cursed every fold and roll and stretch mark because they were all reminders about how my body had failed me by failing to protect my baby in what should have been the safest environment in the world.

I needed something to save me from the negativity and numbness and sadness. I knew I would feel those things; I knew there would be something missing forever, but I also knew that the pain would become manageable, and it would not plague me during every minute of every day forever. The passage of time had already showed me that I had the capacity to feel better. Little things changed: a genuine smile here, the use of an exclamation mark there, the ability to respond to a typed message of support, the ability to hold a conversation over the phone, and then in person.

My sister asked if she could fly out to visit us. I asked her to bring the whole family; if her kids came, they could play with mine and it would be about family and future and love, instead of loss, and insurmountable grief, and wells of tears. She and her husband, and their two wonderful children, would arrive ten days after our tragedy. Once the plans were set, I worried I would be too overwhelmed. There was so much potential for it to be disastrous. But once they arrived, it felt healing and heartwarming to have them with us.

The fundraiser held by our friend afforded us time to spend and gave us the ability to do fun things with the kids; we made the trip about them. We planned a day at the beach, a day at the farm, and a day at the zoo (that turned into a broken-down car and a couple of hours at the park as a consolation prize). There were tears but there were shoulders to cry on. There were empty arms but they were filled by hugs. Cole was missing in everything we did but the presence of all the children, all playing together, was a reminder to focus on what we still had and not solely on what we had lost. No matter our loss and our pain, we also knew that there would always be others who would go through more loss and pain than we had experienced; and so we were also thankful that the devastation of what we were going through had not been worse.

My sister had just recently experienced two traumas herself: a surgery that had a profound, psychological impact on her, and, just as she felt she was returning to her normal self, her daughter was hit by a truck. It literally knocked the vivacious six-year-old out of her boots and flung her ten feet down the road. Miraculously, she only suffered from some scrapes and bruises and a mild concussion. It could have been infinitely worse, and that realization was difficult to process, for all of us. My sister was given a diffuser necklace in which she placed various oils to help promote peace, calmness, emotional healing, acceptance, etc. When she came to visit us, she let me borrow her necklace to help me cope with my own trauma. When I tried to return it to her before they left for home, she gave it to me, along with a bottle of the oil that I had found most helpful (white angelica). After she returned home, I drew a great amount of strength from it, not just from the oil, but from the gift itself; it was something that had meant so much to her and helped her through the most challenging moments in her life – the love she felt for me had moved her to give it to me. In wearing the necklace, I was calmed by the oil and bolstered by my sister's compassion, understanding, kindness, and love.

In the aftermath, in the struggle to keep moving forward, there were nightmares. But they were not nightmares like one might think: reliving the painful moments over and over in my sleep (I suffered enough of that through my waking hours). The nightmares were more cryptic: frightening images accompanied by intense emotions that didn't make immediate sense. They were my mind's attempt at finding logic in what I had gone through, trying to reconcile my new reality with the old, figuring out what it all meant, and how I could take steps into the frightening new world where possibility vs. probability didn't matter – if it was possible, then the threat was real. (Christopher suffered from living life through a worst-case-scenario filter due to traumas he had experienced before meeting me. It is a sad, scary, and exhausting way to live.) Thankfully, I wasn't plagued by nightmares for long. I'm sure my subconscious was still doing a lot of heavy lifting, but my REM cycles were left mostly empty for a time, which was unusual for me but very welcome considering the alternative.

When I returned home from the hospital, I imagined Cole's picture on the wall in our hallway. I didn't actually think, *I would like to get that picture printed and hang it there, on the wall;* I literally expected to see his picture on the wall, where another picture already hung, in the hallway just outside the bathroom, between the bedrooms. Every time I walked into my children's room, or left the bathroom, I expected to see that photo. It was never there. I don't know why I expected it, and I don't know why my mind chose that space to hang a phantom photo, but it kept me unsettled, a piece that was always missing, like Cole would always be missing from everything that I would ever do. (You may wonder why I didn't just hang the picture there to ease my mind. Mums and dads don't often grieve and process the loss of their unborn child the same way. I knew that although hanging that photo in that place would have brought me comfort, it would have brought my husband so much pain, day after day. We did our best to be mindful of each other, on the same journey, but experiencing it differently.)

I found that mornings and evenings were the hardest. Lying in bed having to face the day and in the silence of trying to fall asleep at night, when the only sounds were the dangerous and damaging questions that swirled around and around in my head and never led anywhere except back to the same devastating scenes that I never wanted to relive again.

My grief always found me while I was bathing. Every shower I took for a month after Cole's death brought tears that I could not hold back. Maybe it was because I felt free enough to cry there; I didn't worry about damaging my children with my depression; I didn't fear triggering my husband's own pain; I could just let the tears and the water work to wash away a little bit of mine.

I lost my voice. It was perhaps the strangest symptom of grief that I never expected. As a singer, it was a devastating loss. The very thing that I could use to express myself and find some joy again was completely stripped from me. Not only could I not sing but my throat hurt. Even my talking voice was hoarse and sometimes refused to phonate at all. I couldn't even read my living children bed-time stories, for both the physical pain in my throat and the emotional pain the loss of my voice caused me.

The most contradictory feelings I experienced were in interacting with other people. I wanted to shy away, never have to see, or speak, or explain what I had lost to anyone. At the same time, I didn't want people to ignore what had happened. I wanted everyone to know. I wanted to explain exactly what I was feeling. I wanted them to see my beautiful boy and know just how much I had lost. I wanted to tell strangers. I wanted to find people who had been through the same kind of hurt and talk and cry and wail with them. And still, I wanted to face no one.

When I was pregnant with my other two children, I desperately wanted to have a friend (I would have settled for a distant acquaintance) that I could share the miraculous journey of pregnancy and birth with. There was no one. Then, during my pregnancy with Cole, there was a myriad: a distant friend from college, my closest friend from the music program at University, a best friend from secondary school, another friend from high school … the list went on and on. Some of us talked through our pregnancy, bemoaning the discomforts and sharing the joy of imagined futures. After I birthed my boy and kissed him goodbye, the happy news and beautiful pictures of all my friends' lovely, healthy babies came scrolling into view. I was profoundly happy for them, to experience the joy of pregnancy and birth and the love between a parent and newborn, but each congratulation, each heart-expanding offering of sincere love and happiness was a stabbing reminder of what I had lost. Why couldn't I have shared those most miraculous of moments with those wonderful women when my other two children had been born? Why was it now, after I had experienced the most gut-wrenching loss of my life, that everyone was having their babies; all within a matter of days and weeks? Then again, why did I lose my baby at all? *Why? Why? Why?*

Now, anytime I ask "Why?" for some mundane reason, it seems so stupid, because the biggest "Why" of all, that will never be answered, is why I lost my son a few days before his due date. *Why?* In the absence of the kind of solace an answer would bring, I drew comfort, of a sort, from other people's stories of loss, and their inability to answer "Why?" The shared lack of understanding after such loss made me feel not so alone. When people shared their own stories of loss, it let Christopher and I know that we would get through it. After losing Cole, I hungered to speak to other people that had experienced the same kind of loss. Even though I found it impossible to speak about it without crying, it did so much to melt into the hug of someone who understood and just cry together. It shattered the isolation and gave me hope that there would be support to help me come out functional on the other side. I would be missing a piece, but I could also be whole.

The results from the autopsy revealed almost nothing. Our boy had been perfectly healthy. There was no evidence of a prolonged problem that eventually led to his death, so it was most likely a quick end: that was almost a comfort. From a very small and limited study, it was suggested that he could have passed eight to twelve hours before delivery, so possibly while I was struggling with the contract and the printer, or later, when I was on the way to get checked out by Tesa. I could rule out the tuna, and the tinned baked beans, and maybe sleeping on my back ... but there were so many variables involved and the research that had been done was so narrow that it was not a trustworthy guide by any means and so it left more questions and more ruminating.

I suffered from headaches (previously, a very rare occurrence for me). I eventually realized that they were brought on, not only by the grief and the circular cogitating, but because I wasn't properly taking care of myself. I was forgetting to drink water. I live in the desert, and I was going through day after day of barely drinking any water at all. Once I realized the problem (over a month after losing Cole) I started consciously forcing myself to drink enough water and the headaches became much less frequent.

Cole's death embodied Christopher's acute fear of loss and was his worst nightmare realized. In the hospital, after it was confirmed that Cole's heart had stopped beating. Christopher said, "Now it's just about you and me and Bella and Turner." My eyes grew wide with my own fear of what he meant. We had always talked about having four children, and despite the devastating loss of Cole, I still knew that I wanted a bigger family. If Christopher could not come back from this loss, then I had not only lost Cole, but whatever future children I had believed I would have. The loss was compounded and the future seemed absolutely desolate, barren.

Days after Cole's death, Christopher and I were talking, crying, and processing. I said I couldn't imagine Cole being our last newborn I would ever hold. I couldn't imagine that was the last time I would ever kiss the precious little forehead, or hold the hand of a baby who was the manifestation of our dedication and love. It was too cruel to have it end that way. To my amazement, he agreed. We decided together to move forward with positive intent. We knew that if we did not, although we would never again risk those depths of grief, we would also never again know the pinnacles of joy of creating life, welcoming it into the world, and raising it with love.

After a month had passed, I didn't think I was blaming myself anymore but in opening up to my sister-in-law (who had also experienced pregnancy loss), I realized that deep down, I was still blaming myself and holding myself completely accountable. It may have been warranted, but it may not. First, I had to admit to myself that I blamed myself, that I was guilty, and the only way I was able to do that was in saying it out loud to somebody else. While I kept it to myself, I never fully admitted it. Once I spoke it aloud, I was able to think about it, process it, and come to a fair conclusion about it and that conclusion was that I was, at least in part, guilty of my son's death … but only because I was guilty of being human. After coming to that realization, and forgiving myself for being a naturally-flawed human, my day-to-day became much easier; the empty pit inside of me ceased to suck the rest of me in like a black hole. Despite the loss and the pain, I was able to live again.

Either way, no matter who was really to blame: myself, nature, circumstance; it would never change the fact that my son was gone. No answers, nothing, would allow me to travel back in time and change the outcome. Really, there was no getting over this loss; there was no forgetting. I would always feel the lack of my son's physical presence. But once I understood that and embraced it, I stopped looking for a way to change it. I had to accept it as part of who I was. In that acceptance, I could move forward, and find joy again.

I could fight against the trauma and damage forever, trying to forget, trying to suppress it, but not only would I become bitter and jaded in my lack of success, but my energy would be spent negatively instead of positively. I refuse to destroy the rest of my life with misery because I was blessed with the privilege of growing and nurturing a human life, even if it was only for nine months. I wanted and expected more: years and years of love, frustration, humor, fear, amazement and pride … but I am thankful for what I was given, not permanently embittered by unmet expectation.

My illusion of control was violently ripped from me on February 10, 2020. The only way I could try to regain that sense of control was to make the decision to try to create and nurture life once again and to be proactive in preventing tragedies like Cole's loss in the future, not only for myself, but for others as well.

We remain closed off on this subject for so many understandable reasons: guilt, shame, grief, isolation. And in an age where most taboo subjects are being opened up and publicly discussed, miscarriage and stillbirth are still hidden in the shadows and only discussed by those in the circles unlucky enough to experience such pain. Without speaking out, those feelings of isolation and guilt are perpetuated, the ramifications for society of the grieving family are overlooked and, as a result, there is a sharp shortage of funding to discover the causes of such losses, and how they may be prevented. If my speaking about my experience could console anyone, or inspire anyone to push the boundaries of what little we already know, and subsequently prevent even minimal losses in the future, then I will never stop shouting my painful story out into the world.

Loss is part of the human condition, no one, NO ONE, can escape it. It appears differently: the loss of a beloved pet who was truly a family member, a friend, a grandparent, a parent, a sibling, a child. Under countless circumstances, these losses occur and eat away at our souls, some worse than others, but all have the underlying pain of losing what we once had. It can effectively crumble our foundations of reality until we feel like we are just suspended in the vacuum of space, dark and desolate, with nothing to steady ourselves.

Cole gave me the gift of an ignited faith in God. With a new foundation poured and set by that faith, I am creating a new future that is brighter and more beautiful that I could have ever imagined before. And for that, I thank my son every day.

Instead of letting my loss eat me alive, I accepted it, I bathed in the sorrow of it, and I embraced the new person it forced me to become. I will continue to move forward with it and not let its tragic lessons be lost on me. My son's death will never amount to nothing; he now affects the way I think, see, hear, feel, and live my life – and not in a negative way – always on the side of light and life and thankfulness. I make the conscious decision today, and every day, to have God and my precious son be the positive driving force behind my every motion.

Thank you, my sweet boy, for all that you have given me.

Remembering My Samuel

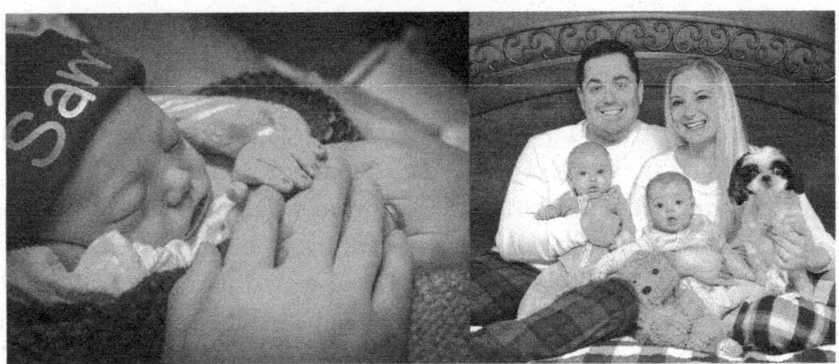

by Rachel Wheeler

We did everything right. Every doctor's appointment was completely normal and every baby check was how it was supposed to be ... until the day before my due date.

First thing in the morning on the day before our Samuel was due, I noticed some bloody tissue in the toilet. I took this as a sign that I was about to go into labor, so I decided to spend the day getting everything cleaned up around the house in anticipation of not being there for a few days.

By the time I slowed down in the afternoon, I noticed I hadn't felt my baby move all day. I thought about it first and decided to lie down on my left side before I said anything. When my husband was finished working, around five pm, I told him I hadn't felt anything all day. He didn't want to jump to conclusions and worry me any further, but he said to definitely call the doctor. I called, left a message for the nurses, and ate dinner while we waited for a call back.

Based on what I told them and that I was due the next day, the nurse said the doctor wanted me to go to triage at the hospital and get a non-stress test. I honestly did not even consider the different scenarios that could be happening. I was just going to another appointment for another test and they were going to check on my baby.

I was totally blindsided. The nurse couldn't find his heartbeat. She politely said she wasn't sure if it was mine that she was hearing so she wanted an ultrasound tech to come in and do a scan. By this time in our pregnancy, 39 weeks and 6 days, we had a pretty good idea of what we were looking at on the ultrasound monitor. As soon as she hovered over his chest-cavity we knew what we were not seeing. His heart was not beating.

The tech turned to me with an ashen face and said she was so sorry but there was no heartbeat. My husband became angry and I went into shock.

The ultrasound tech wanted to be completely sure about what she was seeing, so she had the OB doctor come in and do the scan again. Same result.

My husband immediately started crying, hard. I couldn't feel or do anything. I remember turning to him and apologizing for not crying. I felt guilty that I wasn't weeping, but I couldn't feel anything else. My body was numb. I felt my brain go numb. My chest felt tight. I didn't know what to do.

The doctor advised me that we should get set up for induction and he arranged for us to be moved to the labor and delivery floor. I remember my heart feeling like a lead weight as I was wheeled upstairs, holding my face in my hands. My husband followed behind the nurse in silence. Neither of us could fathom what we needed to do next. We had to call our parents (who were all expecting us to be at the hospital by now anyway), but instead of a birth announcement, we had to tell them that our son was gone.

Those phone calls showed me a side of my parents I had never seen before. They had always protected me from anything bad but that night, there was nothing they could do. They too were heartbroken and helpless.

By the end of our first day of tragedy, I had been started on Pitocin to begin the induction process. The nurse also gave me something to help me sleep. At first, I didn't think I would need it but I quickly changed my mind because I just wanted to get to the next day and do the last thing I needed to do for Samuel: deliver him.

At the beginning of day two of our tragedy, my son's due date, I woke up to find my parents there with my husband, along with my brother and sister-in-law. I still felt numb from the inside out. I had cried a little bit the night before, but I was holding everything inside so I could focus on giving birth.

All day, I was hoping the doctors were wrong. I was hoping so hard that the test was wrong and when Samuel was born, he would cry. Later that night, when it was all over, my husband and I both said that same thing to each other. We had both been thinking it all day.

But the ultrasound had been right. Our son was born silently after only 30 minutes of pushing. The midwife let me know right away that there was nothing physically wrong that she could see. She wanted me to know that there was no apparent suffering he had been through. I remember my husband and I sobbing while the nurse cleaned our son off. They handed him to me and I sobbed even harder with my husband at my side. We spent some time together, just the three of us, before letting our families in to see the baby.

I was so unsure of what to do. I gave birth at 6 PM and the rest of the night both flew by and lasted forever. I cried so much. I remember everyone crying for a long time. Our son, Samuel, looked perfect. He felt perfect. He was the best thing I ever experienced. All the emotion I had been holding in since finding out that he passed away came out and I couldn't control myself. It was the most vulnerable I had ever felt.

Our hospital allowed us to keep Samuel in our recovery room overnight and for as long as we wanted. They allowed us to decide when we wanted the nurse to take him away. Day three of our tragedy began with more crying as soon as we woke up. I asked the nurse to hand my baby to me from the bassinet that I'd had them wheel right next to my bed for the night. My husband sat on my bed with me and we both held our son and sobbed. Looking back, I didn't know it was physically possible to cry as much as we did throughout that entire week. The tears just kept coming.

I was physically cleared to leave the hospital the day after giving birth. We had decided that going home was the best decision at the time because all we were doing was sitting around in a small, uncomfortable hospital room.

When we walked through the door to our home, we both started crying again. *This wasn't how it was supposed to go. We were supposed to bring our baby home.* Instead, we were both emotional and physical wrecks with empty arms.

The next few days run together in my memory. Our parents spent a lot of time around our house making sure we were getting food and filtering visitors for us. Our new, unexpected life had begun and we were just along for the ride. It's a path that must be different for everyone who loses a child. We all have different ways of grieving. We all have different needs. Even my husband and I grieved in different ways. That worried me at first, until I realized we each had to do our own thing personally but we were still there for each other. We never left the other in need of our support. We took this new life together side by side.

Moving forward after the loss of a child turns your world upside down. I experienced new feelings, thoughts, opinions and new people that I had never expected. It took some getting used to but I have carved my path in this life.

I am the mother of an angel baby. I love and miss him every single day. If you're reading this, it is likely that you are the parent of an angel baby now, too. It's hard. It's going to be really hard. But we can do this. Reaching out and finding other people who have experienced the same event doesn't necessarily make it any easier, but it does become less lonely.

At the time of writing my story for this book, I am in my third trimester of my second pregnancy, and we're having twins. This, too, is very hard! But the love I felt for my Samuel the first time I held him is what keeps me going any time I feel scared during this pregnancy. My heart knows what's possible and my Samuel is my motivation for doing everything I can to have these babies delivered healthfully. Samuel, my angel baby, is forever in my heart.

41

Adrian's Story

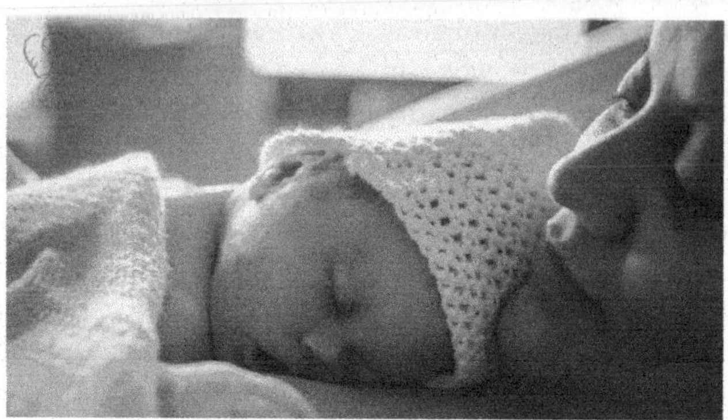

by Miranda Hernandez

I knew I wanted to be a mother since I was a teenager. And I assumed, like most people, that I would meet the right person, get married, and settle down with kids. Unfortunately, that didn't happen for me. After my last relationship ended in my thirties, I decided to become a single mother by choice.

I took some time to prepare before I started trying for a child. I paid off debt, bought a house, and moved into a position with more predictable hours at work. I also took time to find the right donor to contribute the other half of my child's DNA. The process of planning and preparation took years, but it was worth it. I wanted to do everything possible to be prepared.

I was at Walt Disney World the day I got the positive pregnancy test. I had gone on vacation with my sister, and was pleasantly surprised to realize I was pregnant on my first try. I didn't ride any of the rides at the park that day, but I did buy my first onesie—blue, with an image of Thumper. I was already preparing to bring my child home.

The early days of my pregnancy passed easily. I got confirmation at my doctor's office, eased up on heavy physical activity, and started taking a prenatal vitamin. I think the only thing that really bothered me in the beginning was morning sickness. I had the kind where I felt sick constantly, but I could never actually throw up. Those seven weeks were physically hard, but still worth it to me.

The other part I loved from the beginning was writing letters to my son. I wanted to document my memories, so I could share them with him when he was older. I wanted him to know he was so very loved.

Although I was thirty-five and slightly overweight, I was still considered low risk. And so, although my health insurance would cover a hospital birth with an obstetrician, I decided to pay out of pocket for a hospital birth with a practice of certified nurse midwives instead. I also maintained care with my insurance-covered providers, just in case anything developed during my pregnancy.

Throughout the second half of my pregnancy, I continued to see both sets of providers; both sets of providers continually told me I was fine. The obstetric providers recommended induction at thirty-nine weeks because of my age, but my midwives told me it wasn't necessary. Neither set thought to tell me why induction was recommended. Nobody, throughout my entire pregnancy, let me know that stillbirth affects one out of 160 pregnancies in the USA. I wish that statistic were more commonly known.

In my sixth month of pregnancy, I spent several hours in the car one day, and when I took off my shoes at bedtime, my ankles were swollen. The swelling had happened suddenly and it was pretty severe, but when I reported it to my providers the following morning, they weren't concerned. Over the next few months, I developed additional symptoms. I became nauseated again, and experienced intermittent headaches. I also experienced swelling in my hands and face. I reported these things to both sets of providers, but again, nobody was concerned. I now know these things are all symptoms of pre-eclampsia, which happens with somewhere between five and ten percent of all pregnancies.

In my ninth month of pregnancy, my obstetric providers scheduled me for regular non-stress testing; my son always performed above expectation. At each visit, they asked me if I wanted to be induced at thirty-nine weeks. I was tired and huge, but I always refused. I wish they had explained what I was risking.

The week of my due date, I had an appointment for non-stress testing and a checkup with my midwives. At both appointments, I mentioned a sharp pain underneath my right ribs, and that I had been feeling less movement than usual. I wish either set of providers had taken those two symptoms more seriously. I know today that noticeably reduced fetal movement is one of the biggest indicators that something could be wrong with a pregnancy. But neither set of providers was concerned. Both sent me home and told me I was fine.

On June 28, 2017, I was forty weeks and six days pregnant. I lay down on the couch and talked to my son. He was kicking and I was trying to convince him that life was better on the outside. I was ready for him to be born, but I was determined to wait for him to come in his own time. When I woke up the following morning, he had already died.

When I woke up on June 29, I was surprised to realize I had slept the whole night. It was the first night in months that I hadn't needed to get up to pee, or eat something, or just to shift position on the bed. It felt odd to have slept so long, and I felt a little odd too, but I didn't yet understand why.

My sister had come to stay with me for the birth. She drove me to my pre-scheduled appointment that morning. I remember feeling "funny," but then comforted when I felt my son moving during the drive. I realized later the movement I felt was just his body shifting inside me.

We were running a bit late that morning so my sister dropped me off at the front door while she parked. I had been going to appointments so often that everything felt routine. I walked to the testing suite and apologized for being late, but the nurses were all very sweet. They led me to a curtained alcove, making small talk as I pulled up my shirt to apply the testing bands. It felt like any other day. And then the nurse's face changed.

She put the Doppler wand to my belly, in the low spot where we always found his heartbeat. He had been low and engaged for weeks, positioned almost ready for labor. But suddenly she was asking me to move across the room to the ultrasound machine. "It'll give us a different view," she said, trying to stay upbeat.

I think somehow I already knew, but I followed her across the room, feeling silly because there simply couldn't be anything wrong with my baby. We would see it was just an equipment fluke.

She ran the ultrasound wand over me. I saw my son on the screen but he wasn't moving. She asked me to wait. My mind started churning; I still didn't quite comprehend or believe what was happening.

Then a doctor came in the room and picked up the wand. I still don't remember if he said the words before I screamed. I thought, *This can't be happening. My child was just kicking me. I can still feel him. I can't breathe.*

I said the word, "No," but it turned into a scream. And it kept pouring out of me, and I still didn't believe.

I remember the doctor's voice and the nurse sitting next to me. They were trying to be comforting, while also asking me to move. I still think about that moment today, and how every other bed in the testing room was full … and how curtains are not sound-proof. I almost wish I had been present for a prescient echo of that scream, for some kind of premonition that this could happen to me, because until that point, tragedy had always been the thing that touched other people's lives, never mine.

They got me to stand up and walk down the hallway. It felt absurd to be moving on my own. I kept thinking they should carry me. I walked for what seemed like minutes and found myself in a labor and delivery suite. There was a clean hospital gown folded on the edge of the bed as if I were any other patient; as if I were here to have a baby and then take him home with me.

The walk seemed to take all of my energy. I sat on the bed and one of the nurses held me. I cried, and cried, and cried. And it still didn't seem real.

At some point, they found my sister and brought her to me. The nurses asked me questions. The doctor came back with the portable ultrasound machine. We finally decided I would go home for a while and come back later that evening to be induced. I was at 41 weeks exactly. I went home and took a bath, and cried again. I also wrote a long letter to my son. I wanted to document everything while it was fresh. Maybe some part of me still felt like he would read it. Or maybe it was just for me.

We were preparing to return to the hospital when my water broke. Normally it comes out in a trickle but mine was a flood. It was bright red. I think that was the moment it all became real to me.

My son, Adrian James, was born at 3:31 p.m. the following afternoon. And although the midwife had warned me about it, the silence of his birth was still surprising. Babies aren't meant to be born without a sound.

I left the hospital with a handful of photos, memorial footprints, and a weighted teddy bear. I went home with my sister. I crawled into bed and never wanted to leave.

The fact that the body doesn't understand that there is no baby to feed is perhaps the cruelest part of losing a child at the end of pregnancy. I think the only reason I left my bed the following morning was because I was swollen with milk.

I got up and pumped a few drops. I ate and took care of myself because I had decided I would donate my milk. I genuinely think milk donation was the only thing that kept me functioning in those early days; it gave me a reason to take care of myself.

I also visited a funeral home, and planned Adrian's funeral. I was surprised to see not only everyone from my office, but also friends and family who had traveled to be there. Several people spoke at the funeral. My sister especially wrote the most beautiful eulogy. I realized how much my little boy was still loved.

After the funeral, once everyone left, I realized, for the first time, what it meant to be a mother, all alone. I realized that even an introvert could still need community.

I signed up for yoga, and also for a retreat. Yoga was my place to cry. The retreat was my release. It was held in Canada, in a small resort by a lake. The participants were the only guests that week. Only three months after Adrian's death, with the grief still so fresh, it was freeing to spend that time with people who understood, who didn't require me to guard my speech. Some of those women are now my good friends.

That year, I kept writing. I had written twelve letters to Adrian during our pregnancy and after he died, I continued writing. There are 140 letters today, along with a book in progress, and two websites: one devoted to safe and informed pregnancy, and one devoted to the normalization of grief.

I didn't know much of anything about stillbirth when I was pregnant with Adrian; I didn't know I could go to the hospital for what I thought was a routine check-up, and be told my child had no heartbeat. I didn't know, so now I tell people, because these things are important, and this is how I honor my son and his long life that never got to be.

You can read more about Adrian, Miranda, and Adrian's living sister "Peanut" at https://adrianjameshernandez.com.

Letter to the Reader

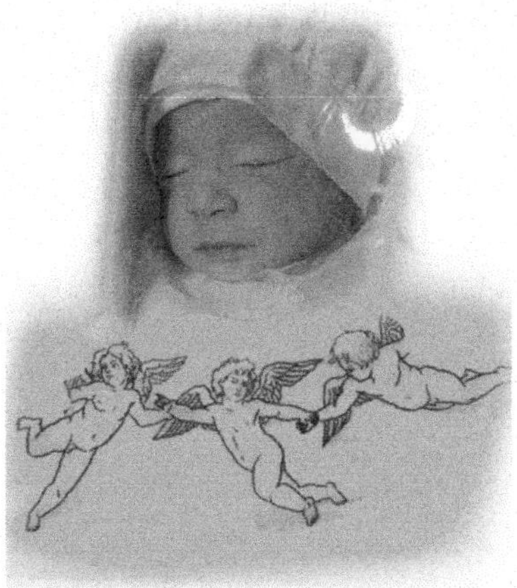

by Kristine Bernadette C. Millanar

Pregnancy is a surprise, a precious gift that so many pray for. No words can describe the hurt I felt when I lost my baby girl, Kylie Brianna at thirty-seven weeks. My world stopped but my tears kept on flowing. I was neither able to see nor touch her. All of our plans for her and for our family were shattered into pieces. Then, my aunt said, "Not all things, living or non-living, will be given to you if those are not part of the Lord's plans. I know it's really hard, and too painful, but you need to accept and surrender to Him for your peace and your angel's peace." Now, everyday, we are trying our best to cope and praying that, with the help of the Lord and our little angel, this grief storm will end soon.

Kylie Brianna, we fell in love with you when you were forming in my womb. Now, we carry you in our hearts, in our thoughts, and in our lives, always. We love you so much, our baby, our beautiful little angel.

Even if we do our best to protect and take care of ourselves and our babies, we cannot assure that they will be given to us. If they are for us then they are for us, if not, we must learn to wait and trust God's process, no matter how hard that may be. Either way, we love our children more than we ever could have imagined and we will love our children forever.

To mothers and fathers who have not experienced child loss: know how lucky and blessed you are. To my fellow bereaved parents: we can share your pain. It always helps to face the day with people who love and support you. Believe that the Lord will not challenge you if you can't overcome that challenge with him. Believe you will make it through the day and have hope that in the future, He will bless you at the right time according to His plans, and you will find a little more balance and room to breathe.

It will be okay in the end; if it is not okay, then it is not the end.

Acknowledgements

My husband, Christopher Fulton, has my eternal gratitude for being my sounding board and supporting me throughout the two years it took to see this difficult project to fruition, even though it is in stark contrast to how he, himself grieves and processes. His strength, fortitude, and ultimate love are blessings that I cherish deeply.

Special thanks to my mother, Loretta Mason, for being there, not only in my darkest hours, but in the years that followed so that I could pursue this creative way to mother my son-in-heaven.

Thank you, Kris Millegan of TrineDay, a dedicated publisher who didn't spare a second in saying he would put these stories in print, for me, for the other parents, for those in need of comfort through their loss, and for the future lives of growing babies.

Thank you, John Lett and Pat Boylan, dear friends and published authors, who showed me such care and love in editing my own story and adding their support to my foundation so that I could see this project through to completion.

Thank you, Tesa Kurin, of Antelope Valley Birth Center, for your absolute dedication to our family.

And Thank you, Teri Martin, the Saunders family, and all our other friends and family, for your kindness and generosity that helped facilitate our healing and this tribute to our son and all other precious babies, lost at birth.

You're Not Alone Resource List

The items on this list were suggested by parents who have experienced pregnancy loss themselves.

Everyone grieves and processes and heals differently; this is by no means a complete list but on these pages, there is a little something for everyone. Even if one idea does not appeal to you, perhaps the next will light a spark of comfort. And even if nothing on this list provides you with the support you need, there are a wealth of local organizations and groups eager to reach out their hand to help guide you through the loss of your cherished offspring; all you have to do is ask.

Comprehensive Support:

- Baby's Breath - babysbreathcanada.ca
- Bears of Hope Pregnancy & Infant Loss Support - bearsofhope.org.au
- David's Hope Pregnancy and Infant Loss Ministry – davidshopeministry.org
- Gathering Hope - Gatheringhope.net
- Hope Mommies - Hopemommies.org
- Leona's Legacy - leonas-legacy.com
- Noel Alexandria Foundation - noelalexandriafoundation.org
- PUSH for Empowered Pregnancy - Pushpregnancy.org
- Return to zero: HOPE - rtzhope.org
- Star Legacy Foundation - starlegacyfoundation.org
- Sunnybrook Pregnancy and Infant Loss Network - pailnetwork.sunnybrook.ca
- The Morning - themorning.com
- The Tears Foundation – thetearsfoundation.org
- Tommy's - tommys.org

Online Support Groups:

- Empty Arms Bereavement Support - Emptyarmsbereavement.org
- Facebook.com has a multitude of groups like:
    1. Loved Baby: Christian Miscarriage & Pregnancy Loss Support for Women
    2. Mom's and Dad's of Babies with Angel Wings (Miscarriage and Still- born)
    3. Stillbirth and Infant Loss Support Group

Angel Gowns:

- Angel Babies - angelbabiesma.org
- David's Cradle - davidscradle.com
- Emma & Evan Foundation - evefoundation.org/angel-gowns
- Kennedy's Angel Gowns - kennedysangelgowns.org
- Rest In His Arms - angelgowns.us

Mementos:

- Birth Certificate – leonas-legacy.com/ll-birth-certificate
- Cremation Jewelry - stardust-memorials.com
- Custom Memorial Portraits – Etsy.com
- Custom Realistic Baby Dolls - rebornbabydolls.org
- Gifts for Bereaved Siblings – Charlies Guys - Charliesguys.org
- Hand and Foot Casting – Empty Arms – emptyarmsbereavement.org/hand-and-foot-casting/
- Knit Hat, Blanket, and Angel Wings, Scaled to Size - Project Robby – projectrobby.com
- Memorial Diamonds - memorial-diamonds.com
- Memorial Jewelry - Held Your Whole Life - heldyourwholelife.com
- The Cooper Project - thecooperproject.org
- Photo Retouching – Angel Pics - babyangelpics.com
- Photos - Now I Lay Me Down to Sleep - nowilaymedowntosleep.org
- Weighted Teddy Bears - Molly Bears - mollybears.org

Podcasts:

- Confessions of a Grieving Mother
- Cradled in Hope/Bridget's Cradles
- Life & Soul with Zoe Clark-Coates
- Love & Loss with Joy Van Staalduinen
- Sisters in Loss
- Smooth Stones Coaching
- Still a Part of Us
- The Morning
- The Worst Girl Gang Ever
- Through the Lens
- Unexpecting

Blogs

- Adriel Booker – adrielbooker.com
- Becky Thompson – beckythompson.com
- Brittany Lee Allen Blog – brittleeallen.com
- Don't Talk About the Baby – donttalkaboutthebaby.com
- Hope Mommies – hopemommies.org
- I am Fruitful – iamfruitful.org
- Saltwater and Honey – saltwaterandhoney.org
- Still Mothers – stillmothers.com
- The Early Pregnancy Loss Association – miscarriagecare.com
- The Morning – themorning.com
- The Uterus Monologues – uterusmonologues.com

Books:

- *Empty Arms: Hope and Support for Those Who Have Suffered a Miscarriage, Stillbirth, or Tubal Pregnancy* by Pam Vredevelt
- *Empty Cradle, Broken Heart: Surviving the Death of Your Baby* by Deborah L. Davis

- *Grace Like Scarlett: Grieving with Hope after Miscarriage and Loss* by Adriel Booker and Amber Haines
- *Grieving the Child I Never Knew: A Devotional for Comfort in the Loss of Your Unborn or Newly Born Child* by Kathe Wunnenberg
- *I Love You Still: A Memorial Baby Book* by Margaret Scofield
- *I'll Hold You in Heaven* by Jack Hayford
- *Love You Forever* by Robert Munsch
- *Loved Baby: 31 Devotions Helping You Grieve and Cherish Your Child after Pregnancy Loss* by Sarah Philpott
- *Ours: Biblical Comfort for Men Grieving Miscarriage* by Eric Schumacher and Paul David Tripp
- *You Are the Mother of All Mothers - A Message of Hope for the Grieving Heart* by Angela Miller

Books for Surviving Siblings:

- *My Brother Lives in Heaven* by Allie Sheehan
- *My Sibling Still: for those who've lost a sibling to miscarriage, stillbirth, and infand death* by Megan Lacourrege and Joshua Wichterich
- *The Duckling In Our Hearts: A Gentle Baby Loss Story* by Kara Mangum and Sandy Sanders
- *The Invisible String* by Patrice Karst and Joanne Lew-Vriethoff
- *We Had To Say Goodbye Before We Even Met: A book for children who have lost a sibling through pregnancy or early baby loss* by Irene Teague and Grainne Knox
- *Why is Mommy Crying?* by I Cori Baill and Heather Bell

Magazines

- *Healing After Pregnancy Loss* – healingafterpregnancyloss.com
- *Sharing Magazine* - nationalshare.org
- *Still Standing Magazine* – stillstandingmag.com

Songs:

- Alyssa Degati – "Angel of Mercy"

- Austin French – "Why God"
- Avril Lavigne - "Head Above Water"
- - "Slipped Away"
- Beth Porch – "You Taught Me What Love Is"
- Beyonce – "Heaven"
- Calum Scott – "You are the Reason"
- Carrie Underwood – "See You Again"
- Celine Dion - "Ashes"
- Christina Perri - "A Thousand Years" - "You Are My Sunshine"
- Colby Grant - "Winterbear"
- Colleen McMahon – "Beautiful Boy"
- Dani and Lizzy – "Dancing in the Sky"
- Daughtry – "Gone Too Soon"
- Diamond Rio – "One More Day"
- Ed Sheeran - "Photograph" -"Small Bump"
- Ellie Holcob - "Red Sea Road"
- Eric Clapton – "Tears in Heaven"
- Eva Cassidy - "Songbird"
- Faith Hill - "There You'll Be"
- Gael Garcia Bernai – "Remember Me"
- George Canyon – "My Name"
- Grace Potter and the Nocturnals – "Stars"
- Halsey – "More"
- Hilary Scott & The Scott Family – "Thy Will"
- Illenium – "Afterlife"
- Jacob Lee – "I Still Know You"
- Jason Gray – "Not Right Now"
- Jhene Aiko - "Promises"
- JJ Heller – "Always"
- Karen Taylor Good – "Precious Child"
- Lady Gaga – "Til it Happens to You" (Tribute to Grieving Parents)

- Leona Lewis - "Footprints in the Sand"
- Lifehouse - "Broken" - "From Where You Are"
- Maddie Wilson – "Wounded"
- Mariah Carey – "One Sweet Day"
- Nick Cage and the Bad Seeds – "Into My Arms"
- Pink - "Beam Me Up"
- Ruelle - "Carry You" - "I Get to Love You"
- Selah – "I Will Carry You"
- Shelly Fraley – "Wish I had the Why"
- Taylor Swift – "Bigger Than the Whole Sky"
- The Cranberries - "When You're Gone"
- The Fallen State - "Nova"
- The Offspring – "Gone Away"
- Vertical Horizon – "Forever"
- VI - "Tiny Angel"
- Yellowcard – "Ten"

EMDR (Eye movement desensitization and reprocessing) is a form of therapy developed to successfully help treat PTSD (Post traumatic stress disorder).

Expert Diagnostic Testing of Placenta by Dr. Kliman -https://medicine.yale.edu/obgyn/kliman/placenta/pregnancyloss/

October is Pregnancy and Infant Loss Awareness Month

October 15 is Pregnancy and Infant Loss Remembrance Day

INDEX
(ORDERED BY BABY'S AGE)

*Gestational age is when Baby was born or taken out, not when Baby stopped growing.

Debbie Martin: Between 4 and 5 Weeks. Unknown. 42 Years. Stay-at-Home Mom. California, U.S.A. 3

Mary Tyler Moore: 6 weeks. Unknown/undisclosed. 6

Rose Skillcorn: 6.5 Weeks. Low Progesterone (perhaps), Polycystic Ovary Syndrome (cause of infertility). 30 Years. Care Assistant. North East of UK. 7

Lisa Ling: 7 weeks. Missed miscarriage. 11

Luci Sorgiovanni: 7 Weeks. Unknown. 16 Years. Student. Western Australia. 12

Nancy Kerrigan: Multiple miscarriages. Unknown/undisclosed. 14

Jessica Oberlin: 8 weeks. Immune Disorder, MTHFR Gene Mutation, Three Clotting Disorders. 24 Years. Clerical Position in Health Care. Michigan, U.S.A.; 7 Weeks. Immune Disorder, MTHFR Gene Mutation, Three Clotting Disorders. 26 Years. Clerical Position in Health Care. Michigan, U.S.A.; 5 Weeks. Immune Disorder, MTHFR Gene Mutation, Three Clotting Disorders. 28 Years. Clerical Position in Health Care. Michigan, U.S.A.; 7 weeks. Immune Disorder, MTHFR Gene Mutation, Three Clotting Disorders. 30 Years. Clerical Position in Health Care. Michigan, U.S.A.; 9 Weeks. Immune Disorder, MTHFR Gene Mutation, Three Clotting Disorders. 30 Years, Michigan, U.S.A. 15

Tabitha Saunders: 8 Weeks 1 Day. Unknown. 24 Years. Mental Health Facility Case Manager. Tennessee, U.S.A. 18

Elisabetta Canalis: Miscarriage. Unknown/undisclosed. 20

Kayla Jones: 7 Weeks. Unknown. 32 Years. School Nurse. B.C., Canada.; 9 Weeks. Unknown. 33 Years. School Nurse. B.C., Canada 21

Sofia Loren: Miscarriage. Low estrogen. 24

Amanda Wong Loi Sing: 9 Weeks. Unknown. 32 Years. Stay-at-Home Mom. Missouri, U.S.A.; 4 Weeks. Unknown. 25 Years. Mental Health Facility Case Manager. Tennessee, U.S.A. 28

Pink: Multiple miscarriages. Unknown/undisclosed. 30

Chelle: 9 Weeks. Ovarian Cyst. 25 Years. Care Assistant. Lancashire, England. 31

Loni Love: 8 weeks. Unknown/undisclosed. 34

Natasha Pandeli-Veyssiere: 6 Weeks. Blighted Ovum and NK Cells. 29 Years. Social Development. France; 4 Weeks. Blighted Ovum and NK Cells. 29 Years. Social Development. France.; 8 Weeks. NK Cells. 29 Years. Social Development. France.; 0 Weeks. Partial Molar. 33 Years. Social Development. France. 35

Ali Wong: Twin miscarriage. Unknown/undisclosed. 41

Dana Colon: 5 Weeks 5 Days. Cushing Disease. 32 Years. Bar and Nightclub Owner. Florida, U.S.A.; 7 Weeks 5 Days. Unknown. 36 Years. Not Working. Florida, U.S.A. ; 10 Weeks. Unknown. 37 Years. Makeup Artist and Cosmetologist, Florida, U.S.A.; Chemical. Unknown. 38 Years. Makeup Artist and Cosmetologist, Florida, U.S.A. 42

Bee Portillo: 10 Weeks 2 Days. Unknown. 29 Years. Stay-at-Home Mom. Texas, U.S.A.... 44

Sergio Portillo Jr.: 10 Weeks 2 Days. Unknown. 31 years. Insurance Agent. Texas, U.S.A. ...47

Mariah Carey: Miscarriage. Unknown/undisclosed. 50

Katie Lee: 5 Weeks 4 Days. Endometriosis. 25 Years. Secretary and Business Partner for a Roofing Company. Georgia, U.S.A.; 5 Weeks 4 Days. Endometriosis. 26 Years. Secretary and Business Partner for a Roofing Company. Georgia, U.S.A. ; 5 Weeks 1 Day. Endometriosis. 26 Years. Secretary and Business Partner for a Roofing Company. Georgia, U.S.A. ; 11 Weeks. Unknown. 26 Years. Secretary and Business Partner for a Roofing Company. Georgia, U.S.A. 51

Alana Zoufal: 8 Weeks. Unknown. 36 Years. Special Education Teacher, Illinois U.S.A.; 14 Weeks. Trisomy 15. 40 Years. Special Education Teacher, Illinois U.S.A. 58

Nicole Kidman: Ectopic pregnancy and a miscarriage around 3 months. Unknown/undisclosed ....66.

Carrie Underwood and Mike Fisher: 3 Miscarriages (around 2 to 3 months). Unknown/undisclosed. 66

Y.Jordan: 11 Weeks. Fibroids. 31 years. Esthetician. Illinois, U.S.A.; 10 Weeks. Fibroids. 32 years. Esthetician. Illinois, U.S.A.; 12 Weeks. Fibroids. 33 years. Esthetician. Illinois, U.S.A. 69

Kirstie Alley: 3 months. Unknown/undisclosed 74

Meghan Markle: (Believed to be) 12 weeks. Unknown/undisclosed. 74

Tori Amos: 3 months. Unknown/undisclosed 77

Dina Mejia: 13 Weeks. Polycystic Ovary Syndrome. 24 Years. Bus Attendant for Kids with Special Needs. Texas, U.S.A. 78

Celine Dion: Miscarriage. Unknown/undisclosed 90

Ms. Khat-Eyes: 13 Weeks. Unknown. 36 Years. Assistant Director for Before & After School Programs. Michigan, U.S.A 91

Tamar Braxton: Miscarriage. Unknown/undisclosed 93

Hailey Shields: 13 Weeks 5 Days. Unknown. 29 Years. Certified Nursing Assistant.

Indiana, U.S.A. 96

Michelle Obama: Miscarriage. Unknown/undisclosed. 100

Tammy Nichols-Rogers: 15.5 Weeks. Unknown. 23 Years. Stay-at-Home Mom. New York, U.S.A 101

Hilaria Baldwin: 16 weeks. Unknown/undisclosed. 102

Dee-Anna Janku: 17 Weeks. Cancer. 26 Years. Secretary. South Carolina, U.S.A... 103

Brooke Shields: Miscarriage. Cervical dysplasia .... 106.

Sylvia Rodriguez: 17 Weeks 5 Days. Quadruple Nuchal Cord. 40 Years. Clinical Research Coordinator. California, U.S.A 107

Marsha Sparks: Twins-18 Weeks 1 Day. Negligence, Premature Rupture of Membranes (PROM), Twin to Twin Transfusion Syndrome (TTTS). 30 Years. On Disability. Kentucky, U.S.A. 112

Beyonce: Multiple miscarriages. Unknown/undisclosed. 115

Justina Engen: 18 Weeks 3 Days. Incompetent Cervix. 27 Years. Stay-at-Home Mom. California, U.S.A.; 12 Weeks. Unknown. 28 years. Stay-at-Home Mom. California, U.S.A.; 14 Weeks. Possible Problem with Placenta (Inconclusive). 32 Years. Lactation Consultant and Birth Photographer. California, U.S.A. 116

Marquise and Morgan Goodwin: 19 weeks. Pregnancy complications.; 19 weeks. Preterm labor and human error. 126

Peter Wright: 23 weeks. Nuchal cord. Mother-44 years. Business owner. Father-31 years. Engineer. California, U.S.A.; 8 weeks. Unknown. Mother-22 years. Homemaker. Father–38 years. Engineer, California, U.S.A 128

Lily Allen: 6 months. Unknown/undisclosed. 131

Lauren Kirwin: 19 Weeks. Car Crash. 21 Years. Nursery Assistant. Manchester, England. ... 132

Chrissy Tiegen: Between 20 and 24 weeks. Pregnancy Complications. 136

Danielle Muzer: 25 Weeks. Placental Abruption. 18 Years. Cosmetologist. New Jersey, U.S.A.; 20 Weeks. Incompetent cervix. 21 Years. Cosmetologist. New Jersey, U.S.A..... 1

Eze Modester: 22 Weeks 4 Days. Unknown. 27 Years. Cake Designer and Maker. Abuja, Eastern Nigeria.; 22 Weeks 3 Days. Unknown. 29 Years. Cake Designer and Maker. Abuja, Eastern Nigeria.; 25 Weeks 5 Days. Unknown. 30 Years. Cake Designer and Maker. Abuja, Eastern Nigeria. 137

Katey Sagal: Almost 8 months. Unknown/undisclosed. 139

Jennifer Coulter: 32 Weeks. Potters Syndrome, Radioactive Iodine (As Treatment for Graves' Disease). 31 Years. Apartment Manager. Christchurch, New Zealand/California, U.S.A.; 18 Weeks. Radioactive Iodine (As Treatment for Graves' Disease). 32 Years. Apartment Manager. California, U.S.A.; 16 Weeks. Radioactive Iodine (As Treatment for Graves' Disease). 33 Years. Apartment Manager. California, U.S.A.; 10

Weeks. Radioactive Iodine (As Treatment for Graves' Disease). 34 Years. Apartment Manager. California, U.S.A. 140

Jackie Kennedy: 8 months. Unknown/undisclosed. 152

Kelsey Kirkpatrick: 32 Weeks. Antiphospholipid Antibody Syndrome (in mother). 25 Years. Travel Agent. Washington, U.S.A. 153

Keanu Reeves: 8 months. Unknown/undisclosed. 156

Laura Ebel: 34 Weeks. Silent Placental Abruption. 31 Years. Certified In-home Daycare Provider. Wisconsin, U.S.A. 157

Annie Lennox: Stillborn. Unknown/undisclosed. 159

Sarah Khouri: 35 Weeks. Cord Accident. 33 Years. Sales Person. Ontario, Canada...... 160.

Jessica Tamez: 35 Weeks 7 Days. Fetal Distress Caused by Intrahepatic Cholestasis. 22 Years. Cashier. Florida, U.S.A. 163

Trinity Brown: 36 Weeks. Unknown. 28 Years. Administrative Support in University Counseling. California, U.S.A. 165

Kristine Bernadette C. Millanar: 37 Weeks. Preeclampsia. 26 Years. HR Professional. Philippines. 229

Janel Neff: 38 Weeks. Placental Abruption. 22 Years. Stay-at-Home Mom and Daycare Provider. Kansas, U.S.A. 167

Melissa Ziegler: 38 Weeks. Blood Clot (that formed for no known reason). 36 Years. Administrative Assistant. Wisconsin, U.S.A. 170

Dustie Euler: Twins-7 Weeks 6 Days. Unknown. 31 Years. Paraprofessional in Early-Childhood Special Education. Missouri, U.S.A.; 38 Weeks 4 Days. Unknown. 31 Years. Paraprofessional in Early-Childhood Special Education. Missouri, U.S.A. 178

Ed Hamilton: 39 Weeks. Malpractice, Breech, Nuchal Cord. Wife-23 Years. Wife-Secretary. Author (Husband)-23 Years. Author (Husband)-Student in Work Study Program. North Carolina, U.S.A. 185

Daniel Harding: 39 Weeks 4 Days. Blood Clots, Perhaps Preeclampsia, and Small Placenta. Mother-29 Years. Administrative Assistant. Father-31 Years. Nursing Home Care Assistant. South West England. 192

Robert Munsch: Full Term. Unknown 197

Michelle Fulton: 39 Weeks 5 Days. Unknown. 34 Years. Stay-at-Home Mom. California, U.S.A 202

Rachel Wheeler: 39 Weeks 6 Days. Unknown. 31 Years. Insurance Claim Representative. New Jersey, U.S.A. 221

Miranda Hernandez: 40 Weeks 6 Days. Undiagnosed Preeclampsia, Placental Abruption. 35 Years. Military Officer and Writer. Texas, U.S.A. 224